Health Economics: An Introduction

Health Economics: An Introduction

Second and Revised Edition

Alan L. Sorkin
University of Maryland,
Baltimore County, and
The Johns Hopkins University

Lexington Books
D.C. Heath and Company
Lexington, Massachusetts
Toronto

Library of Congress Cataloging in Publication Data

Sorkin, Alan L.
  Health economics, an introduction

  Includes index.
  1. Medical economics.   2. Medical economics—United States.   3. Medical economics—Developing countries.   I. Title.
RA410.S64   1983   338.4'73621   83-14911
ISBN 0-669-06917-5

Copyright © 1975, 1984 by D.C. Heath and Company

Fourth printing, December 1986

Published simultaneously in Canada

Printed in the United States of America on acid-free paper

International Standard Book Number: 0-669-06917-5

Library of Congress Catalog Card Number: 83-14911

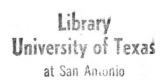

Contents

Figures   ix

Tables   xi

Preface to the Second Edition   xv

Preface to the First Edition   xvii

Chapter 1   **The Health-Services Industry**   1

Health Insurance   4
Manpower   7
Physicians' Fees and Income   8
Dental Income   9
Price Changes   10
Causes of Medical-Care Price Increases   12
Methods of Paying Physicians   13
Health Indexes   14
Distinctive Economic Characteristics of the
    Health-Services Industry   17
Summary   21

Chapter 2   **The Demand for Health Services**   25

Elasticity   27
The Engel Curve   28
Some Difficulties in Estimating the Demand for
    Medical Care   30
A Model of the Demand for Health Services   32
Empirical Studies of the Demand for
    Health Services   35
Physician Inducements: Theoretical Formulation   37
Per-Capita Utilization   39
Summary   41

Chapter 3   **Health Manpower**   45

The Supply and Demand for Health Personnel   45
Methods of Determining Shortage   48
Health-Manpower Legislation   55
The Distribution of Physicians   59
Allied Health Manpower   62

Medical Auxiliaries in Developing Countries   66
Worldwide Trends in the Distribution of
    Health Manpower   68
Foreign Medical Graduates   70
Summary   75

Chapter 4   Hospital Costs and Reimbursement   81

Hospital Statistics   81
Types of Hospitals   83
Hospital Expenditures   84
Components of Hospital Expenditure Increases   85
Causes of Rapid Expenditure Increases   87
Cost Differences between Hospitals—Some
    Technical Issues   89
Hospital Reimbursement   90
Prospective Reimbursement   94
Payment Unit   94
Alternative Budget- or Rate-Setting Methods   96
Some Technical Issues in Prospective
    Reimbursement   97
Empirical Studies of Prospective Reimbursement   99
Certificate of Need   101
Summary   102

Chapter 5   The Costs and Benefits of Health Programs   107

Special Considerations   109
Cost-Benefit Methodology as Applied to the
    Health Field   111
Methodological Issues   114
Rate of Employment   118
Examples of Cost-Benefit Studies   118
Cost-Benefit Analysis in Developing Countries   119
Criticisms of Cost-Benefit Analyses of
    Health Programs   121
Cost-Effectiveness Analysis   122
Example of a Cost-Effectiveness Study   123
Summary   124

**Chapter 6   Health and Economic Development in
                 Developing Countries   129**

Health Programs and Economic Development   132
The Effect of Development on Disease—Some
    Negative Consequences   140
Summary   141

Chapter 7   **Population Growth and Economic Development**   145

Demographic Trends and Projections   145
The Microeconomics of Population Control   148
The Macroeconomics of Population Control   150
Savings and the Burden of Dependency   154
The Theory of Demographic Transition   154
The Child-Survival Hypothesis   157
Birthrates and Economic Activity   158
Birthrates and the Distribution of Income   159
Fertility and Economic Equality—Korea,
    A Case Study   161
Summary   163

Chapter 8   **Health Insurance**   167

Basic Principles of Health Insurance   167
Private Insurance Plans   172
Public Insurance Plans   175
Health-Maintenance Organizations   176
HMO Costs   177
Quality of Care   178
National Health Insurance—Historical Background   179
National Health Insurance—Some General
    Principles   181
National Health Insurance Legislation   184
Summary   190

Chapter 9   **Health and Poverty**   195

Income and Mortality   198
Use of Medical Care   202
Poor Health as a Cause of Low Income   205
Medicaid   206
Medicaid Costs   208
Medical-Care Utilization under Medicaid   210
The Distribution of Medicaid Benefits   212
Health Services for American Indians   214
Urban Indian Health   216
Summary   217

Index   221

About the Author   235

Figures

2–1	Demand Curve for Commodity X	26
2–2	Change in Demand for Commodity X	27
2–3	Engel Curves	29
2–4	Andersen's Behavioral Model of Health Services Use	32
2–5	Impact of Increase in Physician-Population Ratio on Physician Fees and Visits	38
3–1	Relationship of Demand (D) to Supply (S) at Various Price Levels (P)	46
3–2	Relationship of Projected Requirements (R) to Projected Supply (SS) at a Fixed Price (P)	47
3–3	Model of a Monopsonistic Labor Market	48
4–1	Relationship of Short-Run Marginal Cost to Short-Run Average Cost	99
6–1	Hypothetical Lorenz Curves	132
7–1	Human-Investment Approach to Cost-Benefit Analysis of Family-Planning Programs	149
7–2	The Demographic Transition	155

Tables

1-1   Expenditures for Health and Medical Care in the United States, Selected Years, 1929–1980   2

1-2   Health-Care Expenditures as a Percentage of GNP, 1960–1975   3

1-3   Private Health Insurance Coverage, 1940–1979   4

1-4   Proportion of Personal Health Costs Covered by Insurance, Selected Services, 1950–1979   6

1-5   Total Number of Active Health Professionals by Occupation, 1965–1980   7

1-6   Resource-Cost Relative Values Compared to California Relative-Value Scale   9

1-7   Personal Health-Care Expenditures, Average Annual Percentage Change, and Percentage Distribution of Factors Affecting Growth, 1965–1980   10

1-8   Percentage Change in Average Costs of Treatment of Selected Illnesses, 1964–1971: Total Change, Price Change, and Change in Quantity of Inputs   12

1-9   Death Rates in OECD Countries Relative to the U.S. Average, 1978   15

2-1   Price and Quantities Demanded   26

2-2   Correlation of Explanatory Variables with Total Use   34

2-3   Elasticity Estimates, Selected Studies   36

2-4   Impact of Increase in Physician-Population Ratio on Services per Capita   40

3-1   Rates of Return to Dental Education, 1939–1970   52

3-2   Supply and Requirements, Selected Specialties, 1990   55

3-3   Summary of PL 94-484 Authorizations for Health-Professions Education   58

3-4   Number of Students Enrolled and Graduated 1955–56, 1965–66, and 1975–76; and Annual Rates of Increase 1956–1966 and 1966–1976   60

3–5	Number and Percentage Change in Supply of Active MDs for Different Types of Areas, Selected Years, 1960–1978	61
3–6	A Comparison of the Urban Rural Ratio of Physicians by Specialty	62
3–7	An Estimate of the Productivity of Physician's Assistants	64
3–8	Medical and Selected Allied Health Personnel, Various Developing Countries, 1975	69
3–9	Selected Health Workers per 100,000 Inhabitants, 1975	70
3–10	Number of Personnel Produced for Cost of Educating One Physician, Selected Countries	71
3–11	Average Number of Physicians Entering the United States, by World Region, 1965–1973	72
3–12	Number of Foreign Medical Graduates Obtaining Permanent Immigrant Visas, 1952–1978	73
4–1	U.S. Nonfederal Short-Term Hospitals—Selected Data, 1950–1980	82
4–2	Components of Annual Increases in Hospital Expenditures, 1968–1979	87
4–3	Estimated Effects of Prospective Reimbursement Programs on Hospital Cost per Patient Day, per Admission, and per Capita	100
5–1	Total Cost of Illness, 1963 and 1972	112
5–2	Comparison of the Economic Cost of Illness from 1963 and 1972, by Diagnosis	113
5–3	Costs and Benefits of Measles Immunization in Southern Zambia	121
5–4	Cost-Effectiveness Information for the Midwife Home-Visiting Program by Priority Group	124
6–1	Percentage Distribution of Income	131
6–2	Gini Index, United States, 1947–1976	133
6–3	Distribution of Income, Selected Countries	133
6–4	Estimated Productivity Loss Due to Schistosomiasis, Various Countries	135

7–1   Trends in Birthrates and Death Rates, 1775–2050   146

7–2   Current Population Levels and Population Projections
        for Groups of Countries Classified by Stage of
        Type of Development   146

7–3   Cost-Benefit of Family Planning in Egypt During
        the 1960s   149

7–4   Rates of Growth of Real Income, 1961–1963 to
        1971–1973, Selected Countries by Rates of
        Population Growth   153

7–5   Developing Countries in Which Fertility Has Declined
        Appreciably, Selected Years   157

7–6   Estimated Marginal Effect of an Increase of $100
        in Mean per Capita Income on the Gross Reproduction
        Rate, for Countries at Various Levels of Average
        per-Capita Income   161

8–1   Percentages of Persons with and without Insurance
        Protection, 1976   174

8–2   Enrollment in Insurance Companies' Health Policies,
        1978   174

8–3   Ratios of Utilization and Cost Measures in Health-
        Maintenance Organizations to Those in Fee-for-Service
        Independent Practices, Selected Studies   178

8–4   Coverage, Financing, and Type of Provider
        Reimbursement under Selected National Health-
        Insurance Plans, 1975   188

8–5   Federal, State, and Private Expenditures for Alternative
        National Health Insurance Plans, 1975   189

9–1   Trends in Poverty-Income Threshold, Consumer Price
        Index, and Poverty Population, 1960–1980   196

9–2   Prevalence of Selected Chronic Conditions, by Family
        Income, 1968–1973, by Age, Number per 1,000 Persons   201

9–3   Percentage Distribution of Persons by Degree of
        Activity Limitation and Income   202

9–4   Physician Visits per Person, by Family Income, 1964,
        1970, and 1974   203

9–5   Rates of Surgery per 1,000 Persons, Poor and Nonpoor,
        by Age, 1963–1965 and 1976–1978   205

9–6   Number of Recipients, Total Payments, and Payment
        per Recipient under Medicaid, Fiscal Years 1968–1979   209

9–7   Use of Physicians and Hospitals by Low-Income People,
        by Health Status, and by Welfare Eligibility, 1969   210

9–8   Average Medicaid Payment, per Recipient, Whites and
        Nonwhites, 1975–1979   213

9–9   Expenditures per Low-Income Person for Medicaid and
        All Other Free Personal Health Services, by Age Group
        and Area of Residence, 1970   213

9–10   Infant, Tuberculosis, and Gastroenteritis Death Rates:
        Reservation Indians, Whites, and Blacks, 1955–1975   215

Preface to the
Second Edition

Since the publication of the first edition of *Health Economics: An Introduction* 8 years ago, the field of health economics has expanded rapidly, and sophisticated quantitative methods have become widely used in empirical research. While it was possible for a student with little training in economics to comprehend much of the material in the first edition of this book, this is not the case for the second edition. A student lacking a thorough grounding in the principles of micro- and macroeconomics will profit much less from this text than students with this preparation.

Although the primary focus of this book is on the economic aspects of the health-services industry in the United States, approximately 30 percent of the material concerns the economics of health problems in poor countries. While the first edition combined the discussion of the effects of health and population on development in low-income nations into a single chapter, the second edition devotes a separate chapter to the effects of each factor on development.

The statistics presented in this book are the most recent available consistent with accuracy. Considerable disparities in numerical values between sources for the same statistics exist, as do considerable delays in government publication of both health and economic statistics. This reflects, to some extent, the effect of Reagan budget cutbacks on federal statistical-reporting activities.

The entire manuscript was read by Mike McCarroll and Martin Sorkin. While their comments are most helpful, the author alone is responsible for any errors. The several drafts of the manuscript were typed by Mrs. Peggy Bremer in her usual outstanding manner. The manuscript was copyedited by Cynthia Insolio Benn and the index was prepared by William Kiessel.

Preface to the
First Edition

Within the field of human resource economics, the study of the economics of health has advanced rapidly in recent years. The importance of a clear understanding of this subject has increased as the nation moves closer to adoption of a comprehensive health insurance program.

Although the number of students enrolled in health economics courses is larger than ever before, instructors have been handicapped by the lack of an up-to-date textbook. This volume is an attempt to meet such a need. It is written at a basic level, designed to meet the need of undergraduates as well as students enrolled in schools of public health and other medical institutions. While the primary emphasis of the book is on the economics of the health services industry in the United States, approximately one-fourth of the material focuses on health problems in developing countries. Students with a course in the principles of economics will find this book more readily understandable than those with no previous background; however, an effort is made to present basic economic concepts that are essential in order to understand some of the more difficult sections.

Chapter 1 focuses on the distinctive economic characteristics of the health service industry as well as recent trends in expenditures and costs of medical care services in the United States. The next chapter analyzes the demand for health services. Numerous empirical studies are summarized and evaluated. The third chapter is concerned with health manpower. The severity of the physician shortage and the utilization of health auxiliaries in both developed and developing countries are among the topics discussed. Chapter 4 focuses on hospital costs. The major reasons for the acceleration in hospital cost inflation are presented. The next chapter emphasizes cost-benefit and cost-effectiveness analysis. Examples are drawn from both developed and developing nations. Chapter 6 is concerned with the interrelationship between health, population, and economic development in poor countries. The following chapter examines the relationship between health and poverty. Special programs such as the federally funded Neighborhood Health Centers and health programs for American Indians are considered. The final chapter deals with health insurance. The private health insurance industry as well as proposals for public health insurance are discussed.

The author is grateful to the following authors, publishers, and journals for permission to quote copyrighted material: *International Journal of Health Services*; the Johns Hopkins Press for the Josiah Macy, Jr. Foundation, *Auxiliaries in Health Care: Programs in Developing Countries* by N.R.E. Fendall; the Johns Hopkins Press, *Empirical Studies in Health Economics* by Herbert E. Klarman (Ed.); the Overseas Development Council; the *New England Journal of Medicine*; the *Journal of Human Resources*; the American Medical Association; the *Milbank Memorial Fund Quarterly*; the McGraw-Hill Book Company; the Bureau of Public Health Economics; the University of Michigan, Ann Arbor; the J.B. Lippincott Company; and the *Annals of the American Academy of Political and Social Science*.

Rita Keintz, John Owen, David Salkever, Martin Sorkin and Carl Taylor read the entire manuscript. Their constructive comments were most welcome, but the author is solely responsible for any errors. Mrs. Peggy Bremer typed the several drafts of the manuscript in her usual excellent manner. The manuscript was edited by Mary DeVries and the index was prepared by William C. Kiessel. Finally this book is dedicated to my parents, who inculcated an appreciation of learning that shall always remain with me.

1 The Health-Services Industry

Expenditures on health services for medical care in the United States in 1980 reached $247.2 billion,[1] or 9.4 percent of the gross national product (GNP). This represents a per-capita expenditure of $1,067, an extremely high level when one considers that the typical developing country spends approximately $10–$15 per year per person on health services. During 1975 U.S. health-care expenditures were $132.7 billion, which represented 8.4 percent of the GNP. In 1950 expenditures were only 4.6 percent of the GNP. Thus in 30 years health-care expenditures as a fraction of the GNP have more than doubled in the United States. (See table 1–1.)

Among the factors accounting for the rapid growth in medical expenditures are a major increase in the demand for health services, recently augmented by a large rise in government financing; changing methods of paying for health care, including continuous growth of insurance; and the very rapid and continuous increase in health-care prices.

A recent study projects the level of health-care expenditures at $438 billion in 1985, and $758 billion by 1990.[2] Per capita expenditures are projected to rise to $1,850 in 1985 and $3,000 by 1990 compared to approximately $1,100 in 1980. This projection in part reflects the recent historical pattern, in which total health expenditures have approximately doubled every 6 years. The study estimates that total health expenditures will be 10.5 percent of the GNP in 1985 and 11.5 percent in 1990. If these projections are correct, the increases in the share of the GNP allocated to health from 1980 to 1990 would be similar to the gain that actually occurred from 1965 to 1980.

It is interesting to compare the proportion of the GNP allocated to health-care expenditures in the United States with that of several other industrialized countries. The percentage of the GNP devoted to health care by each of nine nations from 1960 through 1975 is presented in table 1–2.

Although of the nine countries Sweden expended the lowest proportion of GNP on health care in 1960, by 1975 it was devoting the second highest share to that purpose. Canada, which had the largest share of the GNP devoted to health in 1960, had the sixth largest share in 1975. Other major shifts occurred during the period 1960–1975; Australia fell from third place, which it shared with France, to seventh; and West Germany rose from fifth place to first, spending 9.7 percent of the GNP on health services in 1975. The position shift for Sweden took place between 1960 and 1965; but those for Australia, Canada, and West Germany occurred primarily after 1965.[3]

1

Table 1–1

Expenditures for Health and Medical Care in the United States, Selected Years, 1929–1980 ($ billions)

Type of Expenditure	1929	1940	1950	1960	1970	1975	1979	1980
Total (dollars)	3.60	4.00	12.7	26.90	68.00	132.70	214.60	247.20
Private expenditures	3.11	3.02	8.96	19.46	42.86	75.81	120.80	143.00
Health and medical services[a]	3.01	2.99	8.75	18.94	40.69	72.74	117.37	139.00
Medical facilities construction	.10	.03	.22	.52	2.17	3.07	3.44	4.00
Public expenditures	.48	.78	3.07	6.40	25.23	56.31	91.39	104.20
Health and medical services	.37	.68	2.47	5.35	22.58	51.35	85.24	96.90
Medical research	——	.03	.07	.47	1.65	2.98	4.33	5.10
Medical facilities construction	.10	.09	.52	.58	1.00	1.99	1.82	2.20
Total expenditures as a percentage of GNP	3.60	4.00	4.60	5.20	7.10	8.60	8.90	9.40
Public expenditures as a percentage of total expenditures	13.30	20.50	25.50	24.70	37.10	42.30	42.00	42.20
Personal care expenditures	3.17	3.50	10.40	22.73	59.13	116.80	189.10	217.90
Private expenditures	2.88	2.98	8.30	17.80	38.58	70.50	113.20	131.50
Public expenditures	.28	.52	2.10	4.93	20.55	46.2	75.9	86.4
Percentage from private expenditures	91.10	85.10	79.80	78.30	65.20	60.40	59.90	60.40
Direct payments	88.50	82.80	68.30	55.50	39.40	32.40	31.80	32.40
Insurance benefits	——	——	8.50	20.70	24.40	26.70	26.70	26.70
Public expenditures	8.90	14.90	20.20	34.80	39.60	40.10	40.20	39.70

Source: Alfred Skolnik and Sophie Dales, "Social Welfare Expenditures, 1972–1973," *Social Security Bulletin* 37, no. 1 (January 1974): 13; Robert Gibson, "National Health Expenditures, 1979," *Health Care Financing Review*, Summary, 1980, pp. 17, 18, and 23; Health Care Financing Administration, Office of Research, Demonstrations, and Statistics, "Health Care Financing Trends," Summer 1981, p. 2; U.S. Department of Health and Human Services, *Health: United States, 1981*, DHHS Publication no. (PHS)82-1232 (Washington, D.C.: U.S. Public Health Service, 1982), pp. 263–264 and 268.

a. Includes medical research.

Though the remaining countries experienced annual increases in the proportion of the GNP devoted to health care, their position remained stable in relation to those of the other countries studied.

Although the data do not permit broad general comparisons of expenditures in one country with those in another, some trends in overall expenditures are evident. The costs of health care have been continually increasing, generally at a more rapid rate than the rise in the GNP. The annual rate of increase in health-care expenditures for all the countries listed, except Canada, have been at least 20 percent higher than their annual GNP growth rate since 1960. In some of the countries the annual rate of growth in health-care expenditures has exceeded the annual rate of growth in the GNP by as much as 50 percent.

Brian Abel-Smith's conclusions about international trends in health-care expenditures implied that the increase in health-care expenditures in industrialized countries would be such that the share of the GNP devoted to health would increase by 1 percent (of the GNP) every 10 years. In retrospect this expectation now appears to have been overconservative.[4] For example, all the countries enumerated in table 1–2, except Australia and the United Kingdom, exceeded this rate of increase in the 1960s. In the 1970s the rate of increase has generally accelerated. All the countries except Canada registered larger increases in the share of the GNP devoted to health services during 1970–1975 than in the 1960s.[5]

In the United States from the end of World War II until 1966, public outlays were approximately 25 percent of total expenditures for health and medical care. Expenditures within both the public and private sectors were increasing rapidly but at roughly the same rate. Considering the public sector, state and local governments were actually spending more than the federal government. The implementation of several major health programs in 1966, particularly Medicare and Medicaid, changed these relationships. Public expenditures reached $56.3 billion in 1975 and thus represented more than 42 percent of the total. From 1975 to 1980 the proportion of expenditures accounted for by government remained roughly constant. From 1975 to 1980 the federal government accounted for slightly more than two-thirds of all government expenditures for health and medical care; the remainder was from state and local funds. This distribution has fluctuated only slightly in recent years, though in 1965, the year before Medicare and Medicaid were enacted, the federal share was less than half as great.

In 1950 private health insurance totaled $1.2 billion. This figure rose to $15.7 billion in 1970, $31.3 billion in 1975, and $50.3 billion in 1980. In 1976 the industry experienced a net underwriting loss of $611 million, primarily because claims and operating expenses for group health-insurance policies was 3 percent above premium income.[6] In 1979 insurance payments

Table 1–2
Health-Care Expenditures as a Percentage of GNP, 1960–1975

Country	1960	1965	1970	1975
Australia	5.0	5.2	5.6	7.0
Canada	5.6	6.1	7.1	7.1
France	5.0	5.9	6.6	8.1
Federal Republic of Germany	4.4	5.2	6.1	9.7
Netherlands	—	5.0	6.3	8.6
Sweden	3.5	5.8	7.5	8.7
United Kingdom	3.8	3.9	4.9	5.6
United States	5.3	5.9	7.2	8.4
Finland	4.2	5.2	5.9	6.8

Source: Joseph Simanis and John Coleman, "Health Care Expenditures in Nine Industrialized Countries, 1960–1976," *Social Security Bulletin* 43, no. 1 (January 1980): 5.

accounted for 44.6 percent of private personal-care expenditures and 26.7 percent of total personal-care expenditures.

Health Insurance

The post-World War II development of fringe benefits through collective bargaining and the growth of union management health and welfare funds have been major forces in the tremendous growth of voluntary health insurance in the United States. (See table 1–3.) The growth of the private and nonprofit health insurance industry was given considerable impetus by President Truman's proposal for *public* national health insurance to meet the problem of lack of individual resources to meet health-care costs.

The data in table 1–3 exaggerate the number of persons with health insurance, since a person with two plans, for example, is counted twice. The overall trend is fairly accurately indicated by the data, however.

In 1977 about four-fifths of the population under age 65 had some form of private health insurance, but the amount and type of coverage was often limited. Persons who have major medical insurance (approximately two-thirds of the population) do have substantial protection against hospital costs, but few have first-dollar coverage because of the coinsurance and deductible requirements of the major medical plans. The remaining third of the population—those without major medical expense protection, the majority of individual buyers of insurance, and those without any private health insurance—must pay directly for a substantial part of their hospital-care costs. If they are medically indigent or live in poverty, they must rely on

Table 1–3
Private Health-Insurance Coverage, 1940–1979
(millions of persons)

Year	Hospital Care	Surgical Care
1940	12.3	5.3
1945	32.1	12.9
1950	76.6	54.2
1955	105.5	88.9
1960	130.0	117.3
1965	153.1	140.5
1970	181.6	162.1
1977	208.3	189.9
1979	220.7	197.8

Source: U.S. Department of Health, Education, and Welfare, *Medical Care Costs and Prices, 1972* (Washington, D.C.: U.S. Government Printing Office, 1972), p. 94; Marjorie Carroll and Ross Arnett, III, "Private Health Insurance Plans in 1978 and 1979: A Review of Coverage, Enrollment, and Financial Experience," *Health Care Financing Review* 3, no. 1 (September 1981): 66.

public programs such as Medicaid to pay or help to pay hospital bills. The majority of these persons were self employed and chose not to buy insurance. However, others worked for small, low-wage-paying employers and could not afford to buy insurance on their own; some were in poor health and could not obtain insurance. From 1980 to 1982 an increasing number have been unemployed or were receiving assistance in meeting their medical expenses through such public programs as Medicare, Medicaid, Champus, the Veterans' Administration, and Workers' Compensation.

Private insurance plans continue to be characterized by exclusions, restrictions, and limitations. They do offer health-care benefits commensurate with what the market will bear in terms of cost and with what some insurance experts consider sound plan design.

An estimated 41 million Americans under age 65 had no private insurance for hospital or surgical care in 1976. In this group were persons who chose not to buy health insurance, those who could not obtain private insurance and had to pay their own bills, and those who received assistance in meeting their medical expenses through various public programs. Estimates of the net number of person under age 65 without coverage by a health insurance plan—public or private—range from 12 to 13 percent of the total group. This amounted in 1976 to approximately 25 million persons.[7]

Because the number of aged served by some public programs is not known, and neither is the extent of the overlap between private coverage and public programs, the number without any economic protection against the costs of health care and illness—though thought to be very small—is difficult to determine. The Bureau of the Census Survey of Income and Education estimates that 3.3 percent of the aged are not covered by any insurance plan.

Once unionized workers obtained basic coverage for hospital and surgical procedures, collective-bargaining agreements began including employer-paid benefits for prescribed drugs and dental care. By 1966 almost 70 million persons were included in health-insurance plans that provided at least partial payment for drugs. Some level of dental benefits were provided to about 4 million. Coverage for prescribed drugs rose 52 percent from 1966 to 1970 and almost at the same rate in the next 5 years before tapering off in 1976. Paid dental-care benefits increased even more dramatically, tripling from 1966 to 1970 and rising at almost that rate in the following 5-year period. At the end of 1977 nearly 23 percent of the population was covered by dental insurance.[8]

For many years the health-insurance industry has been criticized for aggravating cost inflation by its imbalance in benefit coverage. This coverage, which was originally focused almost entirely on hospital care, contributed to inappropriate and expensive patterns of utilization. Since many people were covered for expenses incurred in a hospital but not for ambulatory care, a strong tendency developed to use the hospitals even when less expensive care was more appropriate. Although the emphasis on hospital care has declined, at present nearly 65 percent of all insurance benefits are still paid for hospital-related care.

In spite of the rapid growth of the health-insurance industry, only 44.7 percent of the $113.2 billion of expenses incurred by consumers for health care was covered by insurance. The remainder reflected direct out-of-pocket expenses for noncovered and partially covered personal health-care services. Employer payments for health-insurance premiums are included in this discussion as consumer expenses since the payments are considered to be part of employee income. From 1968 to 1977 the proportion of personal health-care costs covered by insurance increased about one percentage point per year. (See table 1–4.)

In the 1981–1982 recession unemployment rose to 11.3 million in October 1982. Federal officials and labor leaders said 8 million of the 11.3 million unemployed Americans had lost their health-insurance coverage.[9]

Under most health-insurance plans benefits end within 1 month after a person is laid off. Most unemployed workers lack the funds to afford Blue Cross or commercial insurers' individual policies. Not only are these policies more expensive, but the benefits are more limited. Moreover according to federal statistics, the employer pays the entire cost of health insurance for nearly half of all workers.[10] Thus extended layoffs place a severe financial strain on the unemployed worker who attempts to maintain health-insurance coverage.

The advent of Medicare has intensified the pressure on the private insurance industry to increase the level of benefits. The benefits available to Medicare recipients are far more extensive than those currently available to

Table 1–4
Proportion of Personal Health Costs Covered by Insurance, Selected Services, 1950–1979

Year	Total	Hospital Care	Physicians Care	Prescribed Drugs (Out of Hospital)	Dental Care	Other Types of Care
1950	12.2	37.1	12.0	——	——	——
1960	27.8	64.7	30.0	——	——	5.0
1965	32.1	70.9	34.0	2.6	1.5	3.1
1968	34.7	77.2	39.3	3.0	2.4	4.3
1970	37.5	78.2	42.9	4.1	5.4	4.9
1975	43.6	81.3	50.9	6.8	13.0	5.6
1977	45.1	79.2	52.3	8.7	18.8	6.0
1979	44.7	79.1	48.9	9.9	22.3	5.9

Source: Marjorie Carroll and Ross Arnett, III, "Private Health Insurance Plans in 1978 and 1979: A Review of Coverage, Enrollment, and Financial Experience," *Health Care Financing Review* 3, no. 1 (September 1981): 85.

most people with private insurance. The inadequacy of the latter has become increasingly obvious.

The insurance industry is also adversely affected by medical price inflation. If carriers are to broaden the range of insurance benefits, they must raise premiums in order to maintain profit levels. But if charges must be increased 10–15 percent each year merely to finance the same package of benefits, it becomes less feasible to raise premiums for enlarged benefits.

Manpower

About 7.2 million persons were employed in the health-services industry in 1980—in hospitals, convalescent institutions, doctors' offices, and laboratories.[11] About 55 percent of all health workers are employed in hospitals, but in the past 10 years the largest relative increase has been among employees of convalescent institutions (primarily nursing homes). The number so employed rose from 509,000 in 1970 to 1,185,000 in 1980. Table 1–5 indicates the growth in the numbers of various types of health professionals.

Since 1965 the nursing field has grown most rapidly among the health professions. The newest occupation—*physician's assistant*—is increasing most rapidly, having more than doubled in employed personnel in the 5-year period 1975–1980. The original stimulus for development of this specialty was the shortage of physicians and a desire to shift some of the more routine medical tasks from the doctor to the physician's assistant.

Table 1–5
Total Number of Active Health Professionals by Occupation, 1965–1980

Occupation	1965	1970	1975	1980	Percentage Change 1965–1980
Physicians	288,700	323,200	377,400	449,500	55.7
Dentists	96,000	102,200	112,000	126,200	31.4
Optometrists	17,300	18,400	19,900	22,300	28.9
Pharmacists	104,000	113,700	122,800	144,200	38.5
Podiatrists	7,600	7,100	7,300	8,900	17.1
Veterinarians	23,300	25,900	31,300	36,000	54.5
Physician's assistants			4,000[a]	8,800	——
Nurses	601,500	722,000	906,000	1,091,000	81.5

Source: U.S. Department of Health and Human Services, *Third Report to the President and Congress on the Status of Health Professions Personnel in the United States,* DHHS Publication no. (HRA)82-2, (Washington, D.C.: U.S. Department of Health and Human Services, 1982), pp. 2–23; U.S. Department of Health, Education, and Welfare, *Health Resources Statistics, 1976–1977* (Washington, D.C.: U.S. Department of Health, Education, and Welfare, 1979), p. 168; U.S. Department of Commerce, Bureau of the Census, *Statistical Abstract, 1981* (Washington, D.C.: U.S. Government Printing Office, 1981), p. 105.

a. Estimated.

The census labor statistics do not include in the health-care category the more than 1 million persons employed in the manufacture and distribution of drugs, as well as several other occupations that are part of the larger health field. Even with the restricted census definition of the health service industry, the medical-care industry ranked as the second largest employer in the United States 1980, exceeded only by the construction industry. Between 1970 and 1980 the total number of persons employed in the health-service industry increased by 70 percent, compared with a 59 percent gain in the 1960–1970 decade and 54 percent from 1950 to 1960. If present trends continue, the number of workers in the health industry will reach 10 million by 1987.

Physicians' Fees and Income

Standardization of fees in a community has been furthered by the development of using relative-value scales. Such scales assign specified weights to certain physician services on the basis of a consensus among physicians. Given the price of an office visit (one unit), the prices of all other services can be determined. If the physician's usual charge for such a visit is $20, then a one-unit procedure costs $20. Thus if a physical examination is assigned a weight of four units, the cost is $80.

Hsiao and Stason developed a relative-value scale for surgical procedures based on resource costs. Resources costs considered the average time it took a physician to provide a given service and the intensity or complexity of effort involved. Adjustments were made for interspecialty differences in the opportunity costs of training and overhead expenses.[12]

Table 1–6 compares the unit value and relative value for the surgical procedures using the California Relative Value Scale and the Resource Cost Relative Value Scale.

That there is only approximate agreement between the two relative value scales should not be surprising, since one is based on academic considerations whereas the other results from practical negotiation.

The median net income of self-employed physicians rose from $41,800 in 1970 to $78,400 in 1979, an increase of 88 percent. Among the medical specialties, surgeons received the highest income, which in 1979 averaged $96,000.[13]

From 1950 to 1972 physicians' fees generally rose more rapidly than the consumer price index (CPI), reflecting in part a rise in demand for physicians' services without a corresponding increase in the supply of physicians. Growing awareness of the value of physicians' services and the reduction in financial barriers to services through wider insurance coverage have contributed to increased demand. Medicare and Medicare have contributed significantly to increased demand for health care.[14]

Table 1–6
Resource-Cost Relative Values Compared to California Relative-Value Scale

Procedure	California Relative Value Scale		Resource Cost Relative Value
	Unit Value	Relative Value	Relative Value
Chalazion	1.2	0.1	0.6
Diagnostic D & C	4.0	0.4	0.6
Appendectomy	9.5	1.1	1.0
Menisectomy	14.0	1.6	1.2
Vaginal hysterectomy with A-P repair	18.0	2.0	3.0
Cholecystectomy	14.5	1.6	1.6
Bunionectomy	7.0	0.8	1.0
Lumbar laminectomy	26.0	2.9	3.2
Hemorroidectomy	4.8	0.5	0.9

Source: William Hsiao and William Stason, "Toward Developing a Relative Value Scale for Medical and Surgical Services," *Health Care Financing Review* 1, no. 2 (Fall 1979): 31.

Since 1972 physician fees have not risen more rapidly than the CPI. Initially fee increases were moderated under the impact of the Economic Stabilization Program, but since 1974 fee increases may have grown slowly because of the rapid growth in the supply of physicians. Thus from 1950 to 1971 the number of professionally active physicians per 10,000 population increased from 14.2 to 15.9. However, from 1972 to 1980 the figure increased from 15.9 to 20.2 per thousand.

In the postwar period physicians' incomes have increased more rapidly than their fees. This has occurred partly because of an advance in physician productivity, that is, by providing more services in the same or fewer hours of work per week. The shift from home to office and clinic visits, improvement in medical knowledge, the utilization of more capital equipment and health auxiliaries such as physician assistants and pediatric nurse practitioners, and the formation of group practices have all contributed to a sustained increase in physician productivity.

Dental Income

While physicians' economic status has steadily improved, the situation for dentists appears to have sharply deteriorated in recent years. The average cost of dental training and the establishment of a dental practice has risen to $200,000. The high cost of practicing dentistry is making the profession less attractive to bright young people. This helps explain why dental school applications fell to 9,080 in 1980 from 15,000 in 1975 for the 6,000 places in the nation's sixty dental schools. In 1981 some major dental schools were unable to fill available places for the first time in this century, and two dental schools have closed.[15]

The average net income in dentistry is presently $45,000 annually compared with about $60,000 in the early 1970s. This decline has occurred despite enormous inflationary pressures. The fall in dental income helps to explain why there has been a drop in the number of dental school applications.[16]

One reason for the fall in dental income is the 1980 and 1981–82 recessions. With high unemployment and declining income people have reduced their expenditures on dental care. This is reflected in lower dental income and increased competition.

Price Changes

Although the utilization of health services has increased continuously, the major element associated with higher expenditure levels has been rising prices.(See table 1–7.) Thus from 1965 to 1980 nearly three-fifths of the increase in personal health-care expenditures was accounted for by price increases.

Historically medical-care prices have increased more rapidly than the price of goods and services in general. For example, during the 1950s medical-care price increases averaged 4 percent annually —nearly twice the

Table 1–7
Personal Health-Care Expenditures, Average Annual Percentage Change, and Percentage Distribution of Factors Affecting Growth, 1965–1980

Year	Personal Health-Care Expenditures ($ billions)	Average Annual Percentage Change	Factors Affecting Growth in Expenditures			
			All Factors	Prices	Population	Intensity
1965–1980		12.8	100	58	9	33
1966	39.6	10.6	100	46	11	43
1968	50.2	13.1	100	43	8	49
1970	65.1	14.5	100	48	8	44
1972	80.2	11.5	100	40	10	50
1974	101.0	13.9	100	66	7	27
1976	131.8	12.9	100	69	8	23
1978	166.7	12.1	100	69	9	22
1980	217.9	15.2	100	75	8	17

Source: U.S. Department of Health and Human Services, *Health: United States, 1981*, DHHS Publication no. (PHS)82-1232 (Washington, D.C.: U.S. Public Health Service, 1982), p. 26.4.

rate of increase reported for consumer prices as a whole. During the first half of the 1960s, consumer price increases slowed perceptibly. Thus the all-items CPI increased at an average rate of 1.3 percent per annum, while the medical-care index rose 2.5 percent per annum. From 1965 to 1970 prices for goods and services in general rose at an annual rate of 4.2 percent while medical-care prices increased 6.1 percent. The implementation of the Medicare and Medicaid programs, which sharply increased the demand for health services without augmenting supply, were partially responsible for the increase in medical prices during that period. From 1970 to 1974 the long-standing relationship between the CPI (all items) and the medical-care price index changed. The average annual rate of increase for the all-items CPI during that time (6.2 percent) was slightly greater than that recorded for the medical-care component. This can in part be attributed to the continuous mandatory price controls imposed on the health industry for the duration of the Economic Stabilization Program, which began in August 1971 and ended in April 1974.[17]

Some economists and others familiar with the health industry claim that the index has an upward bias because it fails to take account of quality changes. When the quality of goods deteriorates, the index tends to understate the true price rise; conversely, when quality improves, the index tends to overstate the true rise when computing price indexes. The occurrence of quality changes has always posed problems in computing price indexes. This is particularly true with prices for medical care and health services, because quality changes are especially difficult to measure, partly because of advances in medical technology. As a result the view is frequently expressed that the medical-care price index may overstate the actual increase in medical-care prices over time.

Another limitation is the inability of some items to be representative of the total service or commodity. For example, the CPI includes the 15 drugs that have declined slightly in price in recent years. However, newer, more expensive drugs are not included in the index.

As indicated previously, some economists have argued that the medical care price index may overstate the rise in the real cost of health services. Scitovsky and McCall undertook extensive research to test the criticism that the CPI overstates the true price increase because of failure to take account of improvements in the quality of medical services. If this criticism were correct, a more valid measure could be obtained by calculating changes in the total cost of treating specified episodes of illness. Scitovsky and McCall measured changes in the cost of treatment of several medical conditions from 1964 to 1971, breaking cost increases into the components of price changes and input changes.[18] (See table 1–8.)

As indicated in table 1–7, in six cases total cost increases exceeded price increases, while in five cases price increases exceeded cost increases. Thus,

Table 1–8

Percentage Change in Average Costs of Treatment of Selected Illnesses, 1964–1971: Total Change, Price Change, and Change in Quantity of Inputs

Condition	Total	Price	Input
Otitis media (children)	37	32	4
Appendicitis			
Simple	80	76	2
Perforated	115	89	14
Maternity care	56	70	−8
Cancer of the breast	57	66	−5
Forearm fractures (children)			
Cast only	17	14	3
Closed reduction,			
no general anesthetic	102	64	23
Closed Reduction, general			
or regional anesthetic	43	57	−9
Myocardial infarction	126	70	133
Pneumonia (nonhospitalized)	13	32	−14
Duodenal ulcer			
(nonhospitalized)	17	33	−12

Source: Ann Scitovsky and Nelda McCall, *Changes in the Cost of Treatment of Selected Illnesses, 1951–1964–1971*, National Center for Health Services Research, 1976), Research Digest Series, DHEW Publication no. (HRA)77–3161 (Washington, D.C.: U.S. Department of Health, Education, and Welfare, p. 9.

there is no clear indication that as a whole there is an upward or downward bias in the medical care price index.

From 1975 to 1980 overall price inflation has been a major economic problem not only in the United States but most other industrialized countries. From 1975 to 1980 both the medical-care price index and the CPI (all items) have increased at approximately the same rate.

Hospital room rates have experienced the greatest increase in price, with room rates 3.2 times as great in 1980 as compared to 1967. From 1950 to 1980 hospital room rates increased over 1,400 percent. By contrast the prices of prescription drugs were nearly stable from 1950 to 1975, but increased slightly more than 7 percent per year from 1975 to 1980.

Causes of Medical-Care Price Increases

There are a number of important factors associated with the increase in medical-care prices. Wage increases, the growth of health insurance, the relative shortage of some categories of health-care providers, and the utilization of highly sophisticated medical equipment have all contributed to medical-price inflation.[19]

Although some categories of hospital personnel still receive fairly low wages when compared to other persons with similar levels of education and training, their earnings have risen rapidly, especially since 1965. Since hospital productivity has increased more slowly than wages, this has been one factor causing a rapid rise in hospital costs. When wage increases exceed gains in productivity, prices will tend to increase. The upward pressure on wages has been enhanced by the unionization movement among hospital workers. Thus by 1982, roughly one-third of all hospital workers were unionized. Moreover nonunion hospitals will raise wages in order to deter unionization (the threat effect). This kind of inflation is known as *cost-push inflation*, since it originates with higher operating costs for the seller or provider of services, costs that must be passed on to the consumer in the form of price increases in order for the provider to protect his profit margin.

Demand-pull inflation results from an increase in demand that creates a relative shortage of the commodity at constant prices. The price of the commodity is raised in order to bring supply and demand into equilibrium. This concept is very useful for explaining a portion of medical-care price inflation. The increase in consumers' income and the expansion of health insurance (including Medicare), as well as the growth in subsidized health services for the poor (Medicaid), have at times increased the demand for services more rapidly than the quantity supplied resulting in higher prices for health services as the market attempts to restore equilibrium.

Another source of higher medical-care prices is increased use of extremely expensive technology and equipment. Since one objective of hospitals is to maximize the quality of care that is provided, hospital administrators frequently seek to acquire the most sophisticated equipment available, regardless of its potential degree of utilization. Unless the equipment is intensively utilized, however, its cost cannot be amortized over a large number of patients with only modest increase in charges. Thus if the equipment is frequently idle, the cost per person utilizing the equipment is high and charges are increased accordingly. Certificate-of-need regulations, which require hospitals to obtain permission from a local planning authority before undertaking large-scale capital expenditures, attempt to regulate this phase of hospital-cost inflation.

Methods of Paying Physicians

There are basically three different methods of compensating physicians for their services. These are fee-for-service, capitation, and salary. Each of these will be discussed in turn.

The *fee-for-service* approach indicates that the doctor is paid on the basis of each service or activity performed. Thus the physician's net income is based on the total quantity of services rendered minus the costs necessary to render that service. This method of compensating physicians is frequently criticized because it may encourage some physicians to provide excessive care in order to augment their income. Moreover outside of a group-practice setting it may discourage referral to other practitioners, because this would mean the loss of a fee. Thus general practitioners may be providing treatment, when in fact the patient should be referred to a specialist. Another possible outcome is the practice of fee splitting, whereby one physician gets part of a second physician's fee after the former has referred a patient to the latter. Fee splitting is generally considered unethical.

The *capitation* method indicates that a physician is paid a specific amount for each patient that he cares for as opposed to fee-for-service, where the physician is compensated for each specific service rendered. The British National Health Service compensates its participating general practitioners in this manner. Each physician is paid a specific amount per year for each person or family registered with that physician. Thus total income depends on the number of persons for whom the physician is obligated to care rather than the total volume of services rendered. As a result there is no incentive to provide unnecessary treatment, but some critics of this method of compensating physicians believe it results in unnecessary referrals,[20] particularly with the more time consuming or potentially complex cases.

The *salary* method of compensating physicians is similar to the capitation approach in that there is no incentive to overtreat the patient. In the U.S. physicians employed by health-maintenance organizations (HMOs) are often compensated on a salary basis, as are some physicians who are employed in large group practices. In developing countries most of the physicians who are employed in health centers or other government health facilities are salaried, but many frequently are also engaged in private practice, where compensation is obtained on a fee-for-service basis.

The main inducement to the provision of high-quality care, when compensated by salary, is peer pressure. Thus the inducement to good performance depends upon the organized framework in which the doctor functions rather than the method of compensation. As in other occupations, however, low salaries tend to reduce morale with some loss in efficiency.

Health Indexes

Although the health-services industry can be characterized in terms of the industry inputs, it is generally evaluated in terms of industry output. One measure of the output or effectiveness of the health industry is specific indicators of health levels, such as mortality rates, either age-specific or age-adjusted. The advantage of utilizing mortality rates for this purpose is that they can be objectively determined and are readily available in considerable detail for most countries. The quality of the data is sufficient to use for comparisons over time within a country and at a moment of time between nations.

Public health professionals put considerable emphasis on mortality comparisons for making judgments about the relative health levels of particular subpopulations such as young or elderly persons, whites and blacks, or the foreign born versus native born. Thus the success of a nation's medical system is not determined by examining medical inputs, whether manpower or facilities, but by considering the mortality statistics (outputs) of the country in comparison to other nations' at a similar stage of economic development.

Differences within the United States are still considerable. For example in 1979 the infant-mortality rate for blacks was nearly double the rate for whites. The age-adjusted death rate for those living in poverty areas of U.S. center cities is at least 40 percent greater than for high-income residents.

Comparing the United States with other developed countries, the differences are even greater. (See table 1–9.)

For males 45 to 54 (the age group at which earnings are maximized), the United States has the highest death rate of any country in the Organization

Table 1–9
Death Rates In OECD Countries Relative to the U.S. Average, 1978

Country	Infant Mortality	Mortality, Males 45–54	Mortality, Females 45–54
United States	100	100	100
Iceland	83	52	63
Netherlands	71	68	73
Norway	63	71	63
Sweden	57	70	69
Greece	142	58	58
Denmark	65	76	95
Canada	91	88	83
Switzerland	63	70	68
France	78	—	—
Italy	130	87	78
Belgium	102	—	—
United Kingdom	101	107	122
Spain	111	78	73
West Germany	108	89	87
Luxembourg	60	98	85
Ireland	115	—	—
Austria	110	101	84
Japan	62	64	63

Source: World Health Organization Annual, vol. I, Vital Statistics and Causes of Death (Geneva, Switzerland: World Health Organization, 1980), pp. 14–20 and 60–316.

of Economic Cooperation and Development (OECD), with the exception of Great Britain, and has a rate that is nearly double that of some of the member countries.

Although the United States is among the top dozen nations of the world in per-capita income, its infant-mortality rate is much greater than that of a number of countries in Western Europe and Japan, which have much lower per-capita incomes. Moreover the difference between the infant-mortality rate in the United States and most of the countries indicated in table 1–9 *widened* between 1960 and 1978. These major differences in death rates may imply serious deficiencies in the U.S. health system.

In recent years there have been a number of suggestions for better health indices that combine morbidity and mortality data. One interesting approach suggested by B.S. Sanders consists of calculating years of "effective" life expectancy based on mortality and morbidity rates.[21] The index measures the number of years a person is expected to live and be well enough to fulfill a role appropriate to his or her sex and age. This avoids the problem of interpreting measures of disease prevalence by measuring the effects of disease rather than the existence of disease. The determination of these percentage weights is one of the most difficult problems to be considered in constructing a health index.

Chen has developed a health-status index to determine health-program priorities. It is a function of four components: the crude mortality rate in the target population, the crude mortality rate in the reference population, the difference between the observed and expected number of years lost in the target population from mortality, and the difference between the observed and expected number of years lost in the target population from morbidity.[22] This index should not be used in isolation from professional judgment. Thus other factors than the severity of disease impact may affect this index. For example, the number of hospital days and clinic visits is generally taken as *prima facie* evidence of the extent of disease-specific morbidity among the target population, but on closer examination this evidence may be misleading. If a new clinic or hospital were opened in a region where none previously existed, it is possible that many people who would ordinarily stay home because of a particular illness would use the facility, but the resultant increase in clinic visits or hospital days would not be reflective of an increase in the severity of this particular illness.[23]

A health-status index should cover a sufficiently broad range of diseases and conditions having significant impact on the health of the population, and in its disaggregated form it should contribute to analysis between disease-specific input components.

Regardless of how well an index performs in a mathematical sense, it will not be used for program management unless it has practical applicability. Suggested applications for a health-status index are as follows:[24]

1. Determination of priorities for health programs. Such determinations usually imply the ability to differentiate between geographic areas, social groups, morbidity causing conditions, and, of growing importance, consumer preferences.
2. Evaluation of health-services impact. To be useful the health-status index must be highly sensitive to changes in the health of a population over time. These can be reflected in either variations in relative magnitude or relative severity of the illness or shifts within the age distribution of those affected persons.
3. Allocation of resources or assignment of funding levels to various health programs. Funding is not solely a function of health priorities or seriousness of health problems. It may also be dependent on the cost and effectiveness of a program and on its acceptance by both consumers and providers. An index that allows for such factors has greater usefulness for the administrator.

Distinctive Economic Characteristics of the Health-Services Industry

The health industry has a number of unusual dimensions that render inapplicable many of the standard economic principles generally associated with firms and consumers who sell and purchase goods in competitive markets. While various industries may exhibit one or more of these characteristics, the health industry is unique in that all of them apply.

Consumer Ignorance

Very few industries exist where the consumer is as dependent upon the producer for information concerning the quality of the product as in the health-services industry. Generally the consumer is also heavily influenced by the provider's advice concerning the quantity of health services to be purchased.

Limitations on advertising by physicians and dentists, as well as pharmacists in terms of the prices of prescription drugs, have been significantly reduced in recent years.[25] Whether this has resulted in a better-informed public and concomitantly more price competition is an important and unanswered research question. However, a study of variations in restrictions on advertising by optometrists and opticians found that prices were substantially lower in states that permitted advertising.[26]

Restrictions on Entry

Probably the most obvious and most significant interference with competition in the market for physicians' services is the barrier to entry imposed by compulsory licensure. The primary argument in favor of licensing physicians is that the consumer is a poor judge of the quality of medical care and therefore needs assistance concerning the qualifications of those desiring to provide such care. Assuming this to be true, the need for guidance regarding provider qualifications could be met by voluntary *certification* rather than compulsory licensure, however.

The principal objection to such an approach is that some patients might receive bad treatment at the hands of unqualified practitioners who lacked certification. The chief advantage of such a system is greater availability of care and lower prices. For certain health-care needs, practitioners with fewer qualifications than those that physicians possess would clearly be sufficient.

Another example of entry restrictions is the system of limiting hospital privileges to particular physicians. This has been justified in terms of the desire to ensure quality of care (in the institution) and as a way of obtaining free services from participating physicians. It can also be viewed in an economic context as a way of limiting competition and raising the income of hospital physicians. As Kenneth Arrow has observed, "codes of professional ethics, which arise out of the principal-agent relation and afford protection to the principals, can also serve as a cloak for monopoly by the agents."[27]

The Need for Medical Care

The position is frequently taken that health services should be distributed according to need rather than effective economic demand (willingness and ability to pay). Because of the great advances in scientific medicine, health and medical care are now often considered the fourth human necessity, ranking after food, clothing, and shelter. To the extent that society agrees to subsidize the provision of medical care, the incentive for households to provide for health care from their own resources (as through voluntary insurance) is reduced. Those lacking insurance and especially those who prior to their illness could have afforded to pay the normal premium, become in effect freeloaders on the rest of society.

Moreover the amount of public funds available for health programs is limited. Not only do choices have to be made in regard to which health programs should be encouraged, but other sectors of the economy have legitimate claims on public funds. Programs of public safety or crime prevention, skills training for the unemployed, or compensatory education programs may be deemed worthy of public support. A particular public program (health or otherwise) may be justified not because it is necessary or good but because it constitutes a more efficient use of resources than some alternative program.

One major argument advanced in favor of compulsory insurance is that it overcomes the problem of adverse selection. If insurance is completely voluntary, it may be impractical to adjust each household's premium to its expected utilization of health services. To the extent that uniform premiums are charged, however, households with lower than average expected utilization have an incentive to cancel their policies, and this process could continue until the plan collapses.[28]

Externalities

An externality exists when the actions taken by an individual household or firm impose costs or provide benefits on other households or firms, and where no feasible way exists of compensating persons for these costs or benefits. The presence of externalities implies that the individual household or firm, in attempting to maximize its own utility or profit, will not make socially optimal decisions.[29] A well-known example of an externality is the costs associated with air pollution that are imposed on others by the smoke coming from a factory. Another example is the benefit to society that occurs when an individual decides to be vaccinated or treated for a communicable disease. If enough people participate in the vaccination program, this can break the cycle of transmission of disease. Health programs that have external effects, such as a vaccination program, have a social marginal benefit that exceeds the private marginal benefit as perceived by individual consumers. This implies that consumers may not be willing to pay enough for the service to justify its production by private producers, and thus it must be provided by government.

Medical research is a good example of an activity with large external benefits, which, in the absence of government support, may not be undertaken by private sector at appropriate levels. In order for sufficient medical research to be carried out, government subsidization may be required. The optimum level of research is reached when the expected marginal benefit is equal to the expected marginal cost.

Chronic Disequilibrium

One negative characteristic of some health-care markets is the failure of price to reach an equilibrium level, where the quantity demanded and the quantity supplied are equal. Some observers believe that the market for physicians' services has been characterized by chronic excess demand.

The persistence of a disequilibrium is a clear indication that the market departs substantially from perfect competition. When excess demand occurs, physicians are apparently reluctant to let the price of house calls rise to their equilibrium level; instead they introduce a form of service rationing. Thus from the standpoint of the consumer, the delay in receiving service becomes a psychic cost that must be added to the monetary price of care to determine the total cost of service.

Mixture of Consumption and Investment Elements

Some expenditures for health services are undertaken merely to reduce anxiety, pain, or suffering. These are considered *consumption expenditures*. For example, the cost of aspirin to relieve a mild headache is a health-related consumption expenditure. However, some health services, when provided to members of the labor force, may render the individual more productive. For example, an alcoholism-treatment program for production workers may reduce absenteeism and increase workers' performance on the job. The benefits that accrue in the form of increased output represent a return on the investment resulting from the expenditure on health services. This expenditure is considered an investment in human capital. In practice it is frequently difficult to separate out consumption and investment elements of health expenditures.

A basic issue stressed in the health-economics literature is the economists' conceptualization of the health sector as a component of the overall economic system. In most industries and sectors of the economy, output is defined as a good or service. Thus the output of the automobile industry is automobiles, the output of the transportation sector is transportation services, and so on. The function of a sector is defined to be the production of this output, since it is presumed that more of this output is better than less, other things being equal. In the case of the health sector, however, economists are sometimes unwilling to make a similar presumption. Instead there is general agreement that health services are merely a means to the end of better health, the latter being regarded as the primary output of the health sector. But health services (hospital services, physician services, nursing home services) are not the only means to this goal and thus a number of other health-related activities (primary prevention functions of public health and sanitation departments, pollution control activities, health education) could also be regarded as belonging to the health sector.

This approach to defining the scope and output of the health sector has significant implications for efforts to assess the sector's performance and efficiency.[30] In particular it implies that economic efficiency should be defined in terms of minimizing the opportunity cost of achieving any specific level of health (for the population) rather than producing a specified volume and mix of services. Consequently even though each type of service may be produced efficiently, the entire health sector may still be economically inefficient if the mix of services (including the health-related activities cited previously) is nonoptimal.[31]

Summary

Expenditures for health services were 9.4 percent of the GNP in 1980 compared to only 4.6 percent of the GNP in 1950. In most industrialized countries the share of the GNP accounted for by health services has increased rapidly.

From 1965 to 1980, in the United States, price increases have been the single most important factor associated with the rise in expenditures for health. Price inflation is most severe in the hospital sector.

While an increasing proportion of the population have enrolled in health-insurance programs, two major problems are of interest. First, in the short run, the severe 1981–82 recession has deprived millions of American families of health insurance. It is hoped that this problem will be ameliorated as recovery from the business downturn gets underway. Second, the present insurance system distorts the demand for health services. Because a higher proportion of the population has hospitalization insurance than has insurance for out-patient treatment, some patients are hospitalized unnecessarily. This puts upward pressure on hospital costs and distorts resource allocation.

In spite of the high per-capita income in the United States, many less affluent countries have lower death rates among infants and middle-aged men and women. This implies weakness in the structure or functioning of the health-care system in the United States.

A number of features clearly distinguish the health-service industry from industries that are more directly affected by market forces. These include consumer ignorance, restrictions on entry, the perceived need for medical care, externalities, chronic disequilibrium, and the fact that health expenditures have both consumption and investment dimensions.

Notes

1. U.S. Department of Health and Human Services [DHHS], *Health: United States, 1981*, DHHS Publication no. PHS 82-1232 (Washington, D.C.: U.S. Public Health Service, 1982), p. 263.

2. Mark Freeland, George Calat, and Carol Schendler, "Projections of National Health Expenditures, 1980, 1985, and 1990," *Health Care Financing Review* 1, no. 3 (Winter 1980): 11.

3. Joseph Simanis and John Coleman, "Heath Care Expenditures in Nine Industrialized Countries, 1960–1976," *Social Security Bulletin* 43, no. 1 (January 1980): 4.

4. See "Costs, Trends, Causes, and Possible Cost Containment Measures," a discussion paper prepared by the Social Security Department, International Labor Organization, for a Meeting of Experts on the Rising Costs of Medical Care under Social Security, Geneva, Switzerland, May 17–20, 1977.

5. Simanis and Coleman, "Health Care Expenditures in Nine Industrialized Countries," p. 5.

6. Marjorie Smith Carroll, "Private Health Insurance Plans in 1976: An Evaluation," *Social Security Bulletin* 41, no. 9, (September 1978): 3.

7. Ibid., p. 6.

8. Marjorie Smith Carroll and Ross Arnett, III, "Private Health Insurance Plans in 1978 and 1979: A Review of Coverage, Enrollment, and Financial Experience," *Health Care Financing Review* 3, no. 1 (September 1981): 56.

9. "Millions Losing Health Plans as Jobs Vanish," *The Sun*, [Baltimore], October 31, 1982, p. A-13.

10. *Ibid.*

11. U.S. DHHS, *Health*, p. 244.

12. William Hsiao and William Stason, "Toward Developing a Relative Value Scale for Medical and Surgical Services," *Health Care Financing Review* 1, no. 2 (Fall 1979): 35.

13. U.S. Department of Commerce, *Statistical Abstract of the United States, 1981* (Washington, D.C.: U.S. Government Printing Office, 1981), p. 108.

14. U.S. Department of Health, Education, and Welfare [DHEW], *Medical Care Expenditures, Prices, and Costs: Background Book,* DHEW Publication No. (SSA)75-11909 (Washington, D.C.: U.S. Government Printing Office, 1975), p. 58.

15. Sylvia Porter, "Your Money's Worth," *The Washington Post*, August 24, 1982, p. B-7.

16. *Ibid.*

17. U.S. DHEW, *Medical Care Expenditures*, p. 20. Controls were placed on prices for other goods and services for only part of the period.

18. Ann Scitovsky and Nelda McCall, *Changes in the Cost of Treatment of Selected Illnesses, 1951–1964–1971,* Research Digest Series, DHEW Publication no. (HRA)77-3161, (Washington, D.C.: U.S. Department of Health, Education, and Welfare, National Center for Health Services Research, 1976, pp. 1–19.

19. Harold Goldstein, "Health and Medical Care," in Gustav Schuckster and Edwin Dale, Jr. (Eds.), *The Economist Looks at Society* (Lexington, Mass.: Xerox Publishing Company, 1973), p. 169.

20. Milton I. Roemer, "On Paying the Doctor and the Implications of Different Methods," in Roy Elling (Ed.), *National Health Care: Issues and Problems in Socialized Medicine* (New York: Aldine-Atherton, 1971), p.127.

21. B.S. Sanders, "Measuring Community Health Levels," *American Journal of Public Health* 54, no. 7 (July 1964): 1063–1070.

22. Martin Chen, "The G Index for Program Priority," in Robert Berg (Ed.), *Health Status Indexes: Proceedings of a Conference Conducted by Health Services Research* (Chicago: Hospital Research and Educational Trust, 1973), pp. 31–32.

23. Ibid., p. 34.

24. James E. Miller, "Guidelines for Selecting a Health Status Index: Suggested Criteria," in Berg (Ed.), *Health Status Indexes,* pp. 245–246.

25. Victor Fuchs, "Health Care and the United States' Economic System: An Essay in Abnormal Physiology," *The Milbank Memorial Fund Quarterly* 50, no. 2 (April 1972, Part I): 224.

26. L. Benham, "The Effects of Advertising on Prices," unpublished paper, Graduate School of Business, the University of Chicago, 1971, (mimeographed).

27. K.J. Arrow, "The Organization of Economic Activity: Issues Pertinent to the Choice of Market Versus Nonmarket Allocations," in *The Analysis and Evaluation of Public Expenditures: The P.P.B. System*, Subcommittee on Economy in Government of the Joint Economic Committee, 91st Cong. of the United States, 1st Sess. vol. 1, 1969, p. 62.

28. Fuchs, "Health Care and the United States' Economic System," p. 228.

29. The firm or household presumably equates its marginal cost and its marginal benefit. The social optimum requires taking into account the costs and benefits imposed on others.

30. David Salkever and Alan Sorkin, "Economics, Health Economic, and Health Administration," paper prepared for the Association of University Programs in Health Administration, August 1976, p. 30 (mimeographed).

31. U.E. Reinhardt, "Proposed Changes in the Organization of Health Care Delivery: A Review and Critique," *The Milbank Memorial Fund Quarterly* 51, no. 2 (Spring 1973): 169.

2

The Demand for Health Services

What does the economist mean by the concept of demand? *Demand* for a good is defined as the various quantities of a commodity that consumers will purchase at all possible alternative prices, other things being equal. The quantity that consumers will buy is affected by a number of factors, including (1) price of the good, (2) consumers' tastes and preferences, (3) consumers' incomes, and (4) prices of related goods.[1]

This relationship described above is often expressed mathematically by means of a *demand function*: $Q = F(P, Y, Z_1 \ldots Z_n, T)$ where Q is quantity demanded, P is price, Y is income, $Z_1 \ldots Z_n$ are the prices of other goods, and T represents the influence of tastes or preferences. For example, the individual's demand function for movie tickets might be

$$Q = 3E + 6A + .08Y + .9Z_1 + 1.4Z_2 - 68P,$$

where Q is the number of movies attended per year, E and A are years of education and age, respectively (taste variables), Z_1 is the price of an opera ticket, Z_2 is the price of a ticket to a stage play, Y is income, and P is the price of a movie ticket. From the demand function one can calculate the relationship between P and Q *holding all other variables in the demand function constant.*[2] This relationship is termed a *demand schedule.*

A demand schedule indicates the various quantities of the commodity that consumers will purchase given alternative prices of the commodity. A hypothetical demand schedule is shown in table 2–1.

A *demand curve* (figure 2–1) is a demand schedule plotted on an ordinary graph. The vertical axis of the graph measures price per unit. The horizontal axis measures quantity of the commodity purchased per unit of time. Note that the inverse relationship between price and quantity sold makes the demand curve slope downward to the right.

The demand curve represents the *maximum* quantities that consumers will purchase at various prices. At given prices they would always be willing to purchase smaller amounts (if lesser amounts were all they could obtain), but they will not purchase more than the amount shown by the demand curve. The demand curve can also be viewed as indicating the maximum prices that consumers will pay for different quantities per unit of time. They are not willing to pay more but will certainly pay less for each of the various quantities.[3]

A clear distinction must be made between movement along a given

Table 2-1
Price and Quantities Demanded

Price (Dollars)	Quantity (Per Unit of Time)
24	0
22	3
20	6
18	9
16	12
14	15
12	18
10	21
8	24
6	27

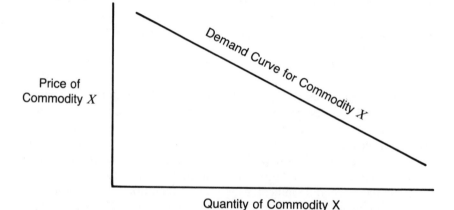

Price of
Commodity X

Quantity of Commodity X
Purchased per Unit of Time

Figure 2-1. Demand Curve for Commodity X

demand curve and a shift in the curve itself. The former is termed an increase or decrease in the *quantity demanded*, whereas the latter is known as a *change in demand*. A change in the quantity demanded results from variations in the price of the good, with all other factors affecting the quantity purchased remaining unchanged. For example, in figure 2-2, a decrease in price from P to P_1 increases the quantity demanded from X to X_1. When the factors held constant in defining a given state of demand change, the demand curve itself will change. Thus in figure 2-2, an increase in consumers' incomes will shift the demand curve to the right from DD to D_1D_1. A shift in consumer preferences to commodity X and away from other goods will have the same result.

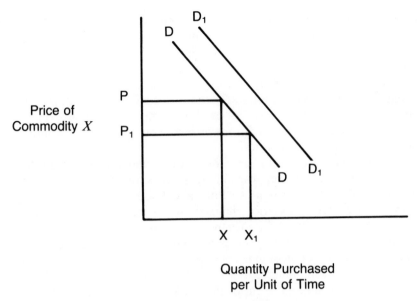

Quantity Purchased
per Unit of Time

Figure 2–2. Change in Demand for Commodity X

Elasticity

Price elasticity refers to the responsiveness of the quantity demanded to changes in the price of the product, all other factors being held constant. Alfred Marshall first developed the concept of the coefficient of elasticity, which is defined as the percentage change in quantity demanded divided by the percentage change in price, when the price change is small.[4] In terms of algebra, the elasticity definition appears as

$$\varepsilon = \frac{\dfrac{\Delta X}{X}}{-\dfrac{\Delta P}{P}}$$

The formula can be visualized by reference to figure 2–2. The delta means "small change in." The change in quantity from X to X_1 is ΔX. The change in price from P to P_1 is ΔP. The number or coefficient denoting elasticity is obtained by dividing a percentage by a percentage and is a pure number independent of any unit of measurement. When the elasticity coefficient is less than 1, demand is defined to be inelastic; when the coefficient is greater than 1, demand is elastic; and when the coefficient is equal to 1, demand is considered to be of unitary elasticity. Three important factors influence elasticity of demand for a commodity: (1) the availability of substitutes for the commodity, (2) the number of alternative uses for the commodity, and (3) the price of the commodity relative to consumers' incomes.

The availability of substitutes is probably the most important factor enumerated. If close substitutes are readily available, demand for a given commodity tends to be elastic. For example, if the price of margarine falls while the price of butter remains unchanged, consumers tend to purchase more margarine and less butter.

The greater the number of uses for a given commodity, the more elastic will be the demand for it. Suppose that steel could only be used in the making of automobiles. There would be little likelihood for much variation in quantity purchased as its price changed, and demand for steel would be inelastic. Steel can in fact be used in the manufacturing of hundreds of items, so the possible variation in quantity purchased is quite large and tends to make the demand for steel more elastic.

Demand for commodities that account for a large fraction of the consumer's income will be more elastic than those that are only a small proportion of total consumer expenditures. Thus goods such as air conditioners, which require large outlays, make consumers price conscious. Quantity demanded is likely to vary considerably in response to price changes. For items such as salt, which account for a negligible fraction of consumer incomes, changes in price are likely to have little effect on the quantity demanded.

The Engel Curve

A demand curve indicates the different quantities of one good that the consumer will purchase at various possible *prices*, other things being equal. An *Engel curve* shows the different quantities of one good that the consumer will purchase at various levels of *income*, other things being equal.[5] Engel curves for two different types of commodities are shown in figure 2–3.

Engel curves provide useful information regarding consumption patterns for various commodities and for different individuals. For basic items such as food, as the consumer's income increases from very low levels, his or her consumption may increase considerably. As the income continues to rise, however, the increases in consumption become less than proportional to the income gains. This is illustrated in figure 2–3A. For other items such as recreation or luxury goods, expenditures tend to increase in greater proportion than income. The Engel curve presented in figure 2–3B reflects this situation.

Income elasticity refers to the responsiveness of the quantity purchased to changes in income. When the percentage change in the quantity pur-

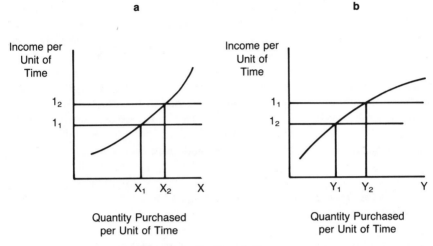

Figure 2–3. Engel Curves

chased is smaller than the percentage change in income, the commodity has an income-elasticity coefficient less than 1. Should the percentage change in the quantity purchased be greater than the percentage change in income, however, then the income-elasticity coefficient would be greater than 1. If the percentage change in the quantity purchased is equal to the percentage change in income, the income-elasticity coefficient is equal to 1.

Traditionally, empirical demand studies have concentrated on three aspects of demand behavior represented by the simplest model: own price effects (effects of change in the price of a good on quantity demanded), cross-price effects (effects on quantity demanded of changes in the prices of *other* goods), and income effects. More recently this model has been extended by the recognition that time is also a constraint on the consumers' decisions and that the purchase and consumption of some commodities, such as medical care, may involve considerable amounts of time (the time price).[6] These developments raise several new issues for empirical research, such as the responsiveness of demand to change in time price and to variations in the value of time (usually measured by earnings per time unit).

The theory of consumer demand for medical services has also been extended by Grossman to include the demand for health itself. [7] The demand-for-health model explicitly incorporates the view that health services are purchased as a means to the end of better health. In this model individuals are viewed as choosing their own health level, or "stock of health capital," with medical care being one way to add to this stock (or at least to retard its depreciation). The factors determining the quantity of health care demanded are, of course, the same as those determining the demand for medical care. However, the model improves one's view of consumer behavior in several ways. For example, it provides a coherent overall approach to the demand for a variety of goods or services, all of which have important (positive or negative) effects on health, such as cigarettes, alcohol, clean air, and health foods. Also, by emphasizing the individual's role in "producing" his or her own health, it indicates that the individual's knowledge enters into the production process directly and may even substitute for professional medical services. Finally, the model indicates an investment motive for purchasing medical care; increases in the stock of health capital, resulting from such purchases, may increase the individual's ability to work and earn income or to carry out other activities.[8]

Some Difficulties in Estimating the Demand for Medical Care

Most providers of health care are price setters rather than price takers. Therefore health-care prices may remain constant for long periods while variations in demand result in changes in rates of utilization rather than increases or decreases in price. This type of seller behavior greatly increases the difficulty of estimating price elasticities of demand.[9] Conceptually, in order to estimate demand curves for a typical individual, one would need a set of data on individuals with very similar characteristics who are charged different prices. The existence of third-party or insurance payments for some, but not all individuals, or the existence of differing proportions of insurance coverage, can help to generate such information.

Because of the unusual characteristics of the medical marketplace, the independent variables (factors determining demand) used to estimate the demand for health services have differed in a number of respects from those used in demand studies in other sectors. Particularly important factors are health insurance, provider influence over demand, and medical "need."[10]

Health insurance influences demand by reducing the price the consumer pays at the time services are purchased (sometimes called the *net price*) below that charged by the provider. However, because most insurance policies include features such as deductibles, limits, coinsurance, or co-payments, the actual relationship between net price and the price charged by the provider may be very complex and somewhat dependent on the quantity of services purchased. Empirical demand studies have not yet been able to resolve this research problem satisfactorily. Instead they have either (1) assumed that the consumer's coinsurance rate (the percentage of the price paid out-of-pocket) is approximately constant and therefore used an empirically determined average coinsurance rate as an additional independent variable in the demand function or (2) simply added dichotomous independent variables for the type of insurance coverage (Blue Cross, Medicare, Medicaid) held by the consumer.

In order to explore the suppliers' influence on demand thoroughly, a well-developed theory of provider behavior is required that can be integrated into a consumer-demand framework. However, this theoretical formulation has not been developed and empirical demand studies that attempt to incorporate provider influence have relied instead on the simple hypothesis that providers will generate more demand for their services when the providers themselves are in more plentiful supply. To test this hypothesis, *availability* variables (such as the number of physicians per capita and the number of hospital beds per capita) have been included in empirical demand functions. In general these availability variables (particularly hospital beds per capita) appear to be strongly related to the quantity of services consumed.[11]

In the theoretical and empirical literature on consumer demand for health-services taste variables have received little attention. Yet in studying the demand for medical services, one taste variable of crucial importance is the health status or medical need of the consumer. Since this factor is very strongly related to the quantity of services demanded and because it is also correlated with other independent variables (such as income and insurance coverage), the inclusion of health-status variables in an empirical demand equation is necessary to avoid substantial biases in results.[12] Of course information on health status is limited, and the variables constructed from the information available have not generally been very detailed.

What is the appropriate dependent variable in medical-care demand studies? One writer has suggested that it is the dollar amount a person spends, since for a given expenditure the physician will provide a certain treatment.[13] However, an empirical measure such as medical-care expenditures may bias the effects of the factors believed to influence demand (prices and income), if it is not first adjusted for price changes and variations in the quality of the product itself. These problems are present in both time-series and cross-section analysis. For example, per-capita medical expenditures are a combination of both the price charged for the treatment and the number of treatments obtained. If a rise in the patient's economic resources is accompanied by a rise in medical-care expenditures, the latter may be merely the result of either an increase in the price to the patient (the sliding-scale fee schedule) or an increase in his consumption of medical care services itself.

Physical measures such as doctor visits or length of stay in the hospital also have their disadvantages. Not only are these variables heterogeneous (especially with respect to quality), but these measures also fail to reflect changes in the state of the art and in medical technology.

A Model of the Demand for Health Services

One of the best-known comprehensive models of the demand for health
services is Andersen's Behavioral Model,[14] which concentrates on individual determinants of utilization behavior. According to this model, an individual's decision to utilize medical services depends on a sequence of
conditions grouped into three components: predisposing, enabling, and
need, as indicated in figure 2–4.

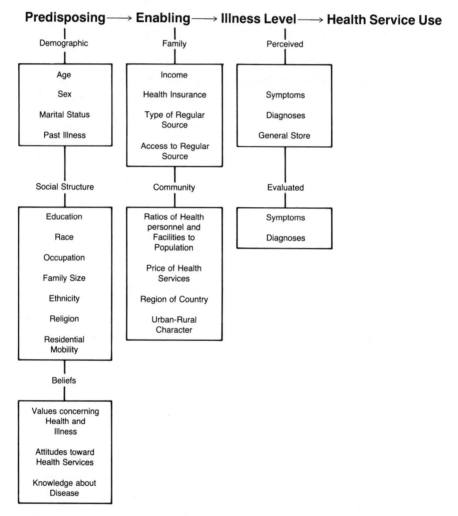

Figure 2–4. Andersen's Behavioral Model of Health Services Use

The *predisposing* component includes variables describing individual factors that are indirectly associated with utilization and are not considered to be a specific reason for using health services. These factors involve demographic, social structure, and health-belief variables. Age, sex, and marital status are examples of demographic variables that are closely associated with health-services use. Social structure is characterized by variables such as education, occupation, and residence that might influence the physical and social environment of the individual. Beliefs about illness and medical care can be considered as a predisposing condition since these health beliefs are likely to influence illness behavior.

The *enabling* component include variables that allow an individual the means to seek care. Enabling conditions can be estimated by family resources such as income, insurance coverage, and regular source of care, and by community resources related to the overall supply of health services.

Given the existence of both predisposing and enabling conditions, the individual's utilization of health services also depends on medical need. This *need* component can be disaggregated into *perceived need* as measured by self-reported health status or sick days and *evaluated need* as estimated by clinical diagnosis. In empirical assessments of Andersen's model, need variables generally have been found to be the strongest predictors of utilization. (See table 2–2.) Certain enabling variables related to delivery-system characteristics also have been found to be important.

Table 2–2 shows that each component of the model is correlated with families' use of health services. The need component, as expected, is most closely associated with use. Families who report the most illness and those who are most likely to see a doctor for symptoms of illness and physical examinations tend to use the most health services. The number of disability days was the best single predictor of family total use of health services, although all the measures of need showed statistically significant and substantively meaningful relationships to health-service use.

The predisposing component represented by the family-composition variables followed need in magnitude of correlation with use. Family size was the best single predictor of use among these variables. Large families, those with young children, and those headed by younger persons and married persons tend to be the highest users.

Income was the family resource best able to account for differences in use patterns. Families with high incomes and health-insurance coverage used more services than those with low incomes and no health insurance. In addition, the volume of services used is related to the family's regular source of medical care. The amount of care used is least for families with no regular source, intermediate for those who visit a clinic or general practitioner as their regular source of care, and greatest for those who report a specialist as their primary physician.[15]

Table 2–2
Correlation of Explanatory Variables
with Total Use

(Independent Variable)	Correlation
Predisposing	
Family composition	
Family size	.24
Sex of head	−.14
Marital status of head	____b
Age of head	−.04
Age of oldest member	____a
Age of youngest member	−.18
Social structure	
Employment of main earner	____b
Social class of main earner	.08
Occupation of main earner	.07
Education of head	.07
Ethnicity	.04
Race	.09
Health beliefs	
Value of health services	.08
Value of physicians	____a
Value of good health	____a
Value of health insurance	−.04
Attitude toward health services	.06
Attitude toward physician use	.04
Knowledge of disease	.04
Enabling	
Family Resources	
Income	.20
Savings	____a
Health insurance	.18
Health source of care	.15
Welfare care	.05
Need	
Illness	
Symptoms	.27
Disability days	.45
Health level	.23
Free care for major illnesses	.10
Response	
Seeing doctor for symptoms	.20
Regular physical examinations	.16

Source: Adapted from Ronald Andersen, *A Behavioral Model of Families' Use of Health Services*, Center for Health Administration Studies, Research Series 25, (Chicago: Graduate School of Business, The University of Chicago, 1968), p. 32.

a. Not significant at the .01 level.

b. Not calculated.

Empirical Studies of the Demand for Health Services

Empirical studies of demand have two purposes. The first is explanation—
the ability to specify and estimate the relationship between use of a product
or service and the factors influencing its use. The other important application of this kind of study is prediction of future demand. Such estimates can
serve, for example, as guides for determining the numbers and types of
health personnel and medical-care facilities required in the future.

Empirical results of a number of studies of the demand for health
services are summarized in table 2–3. These findings suggest that the
demand for dental care and physician's care are negatively related to the
price of care, but the elasticities of demand with respect to money prices are
very small.

The estimates of money-price elasticities of close to −0.10 shown in the
table are important, because earlier studies using less refined theoretical
models and aggregate data report price elasticites close to −1.00. The earlier studies were in error because they were not able to account for other
economic and demographic variables in an appropriate manner.[16]

Holtmann and Olsen found that the price elasticity of demand falls as insurance coverage increases. Thus they found a price elasticity of demand for
physician's care of −0.164 for households without effective insurance coverage, but −0.097 for households with effective insurance coverage.[17] This
is consistent with the Phelps and Newhouse position that the price elasticity
of demand for medical care approaches zero as insurance coverage increases.

In addition, table 2–3 indicates support for the hypothesis that time
prices are important in determining the demand for care but that the
importance of time as a rationing device varies across the types of care
studied.[18] It does appear, however, that time prices become more important
than money prices when money prices are smaller.

In medical care time is used in traveling to a provider and waiting to be
treated at the provider's setting. The following example illustrates how
differences in time costs affect the price elasticity of demand for a service.

Assume that the patient's out-of-pocket price for visiting a medical provider is $10 and that the time costs are equal to $20, the total price of a visit
is, therefore, $30. If the elasticity of the medical services with respect to
total price were −1.0, meaning that a 10 percent change in total price would
result in a 10 percent change in use, and if the out-of-pocket price dropped
50 percent (from $10 to $5), the result would be only a 20 percent decrease
in the total price of care ($30 to $25). This 20 percent change in the total
price would lead to a 20 percent change in use, because the price elasticity is
−1.0. Thus, when an out-of-pocket price is reduced by 50 percent and use
increases only 20 percent, the calculated price elasticity is −0.4. The demand

for that service is thereby estimated to be price inelastic. Thus, as time costs contribute a large proportion of the total price, the calculated price elasticity of demand becomes smaller.[19]

Most of the empirical studies of income elasticity (see table 2–3) have measured income in terms of current income. Yet current income has two major weaknesses. First, it contains transitory income, which will bias the estimated income elasticity toward zero if demand in fact relates to permanent income. A second defect in using current income in this analysis is that it is presumptively indigenous because of the effect of illness on both income and the demand for medical services. Both of these problems could be avoided by using a measure of permanent income; yet there is no standard method for measuring it. Measures that better approximate permanent income (such as use of several years of income) should improve the estimation of both income elasticities and the interactions of price elasticities with income.[20]

Demand equations for general-practitioner and internist visits were estimated from the 1970 National Opinion Research Survey data on health-

Table 2–3
Elasticity Estimates, Selected Studies

Study	Type of Care	Price	Income	Waiting Time	Travel Time
Holtmann and Olsen	Dental	−0.127	0.293	−0.209	−0.077
	Physician	−0.121	0.057	0.008	
	Uninsured	−0.164	0.067	−0.015	
	Insured	−0.097	0.056	0.039	
	Medicare	−0.145	0.133	−0.014	
	Child physical	0.02	0.048	−0.06	−0.01
M. Feldstein	In-patient hospital	−1.12	0.54		
Davis and Russell	Out-patient care	−1.03	0.72		
	In-patient hospital	−0.46[a]	0.35		
		−0.15[b]			
Phelps and Newhouse	Physician	−0.10	0.08		
	Hospital out-patient	−0.13	0.15		
Acton	Public out-patient			0.12	−0.96
	Private			−0.05	−0.25
P. Feldstein	Dental	−1.43	1.71		
Phelps and Newhouse	Hospital	−0.08			
	Physician	−0.14			
	Dental	−0.16			

Source: A.G. Holtmann and E.O. Olsen, Jr., *The Economics of the Private Demand for Outpatient Health Care*, DHEW Publication no. (NIH)78-1262 (Washington, D.C.: U.S. Government Printing Office, 1978), John E. Fogarty International Center for Advanced Studies in the Health Sciences pp. 76–77.

a. Admissions.

b. Length of stay.

service utilization and expenditure. The results showed significant differences between demand equations for general-practitioner visits and those for internist visits. Of potential importance was an apparent substitution of internists for general practitioners as ability to pay (income or insurance coverage) increased. Own-price elasticities were low for both general practitioners and internists but were even lower for the latter (0.1–0.2) than the former (0.2–0.3). The demand for services of the two specialties also differed with respect to disability days, age, sex, residence, and race.[21]

Beyond childhood, use of general-practitioner and internist services increases with age. One can think of age as a need variable, like disability days, and predict greater demand for physician services among older persons as a reflection of their greater need. In terms of Grossman's health-capital model,[22] which assumes that the rate of health-capital depreciation increases with age beyond some point in the life cycle, older persons purchase more services to increase their production of gross investment in health capital and thereby offset part of the reduction in their health capital caused by the greater rate of depreciation.

Grossman has argued that an increase in human capital as measured by education, improves efficiency in the production of health. Hence the better educated are able to produce greater amounts of gross investment in health capital with given levels of direct inputs and have an incentive to offset part of the increase in health by reducing their purchase of physician services. However, the evidence to date contradicts this hypothesis, and other things being equal, physician utilization increases with education.

Physician Inducements: Theoretical Formulation

Neoclassical theory argues that the market for physician services acts like any normally functioning market. When the supply of physicians' services increases from S_1 to S_2 (figure 2–5), individual workloads fall, as a fixed patient load is spread among more physicians. Physicians' incomes consequently decline. Physicians respond to this increased competition by reducing their fees from P_a to P_b, and the demand for physicians' services increases at this new (lower) price. Visits increase from V_a to V_b (note that the original demand curve (D_1) is not changed).

An increase in the number of physicians will also increase utilization by lowering the time price of care.[23] Thus greater access to physicians presumably reduces travel distances as well as waiting time in the physician's office.

As the physician-population ratio rises, individual workloads fall, and so do physicians' incomes. Under the inducement hypothesis, however, market equilibrium can be obtained not only by adjustments in price, but also by influencing the consumer's perception of need. Physicians may

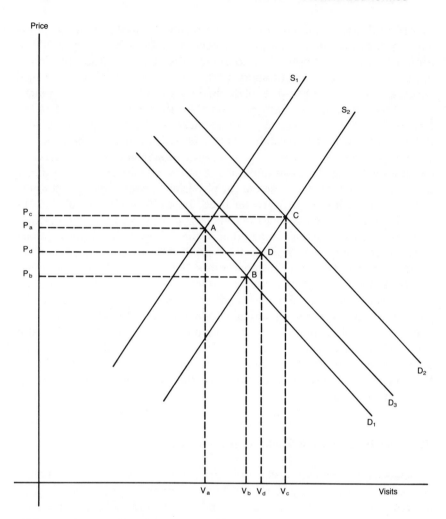

Figure 2–5. Impact of Increase in Physician-Population Ratio on Physicians' Fees and Visits

respond to this change by generating greater demand for their services. They may either increase their output or raise their fees, or both. In figure 2–5 the demand curve is shifted upward from D_1 to D_2. In this case both utilization (from V_a to V_c) and price (from P_a to P_c) have increased, and the ability of the provider to increase demand is demonstrated. Individual physicians' workloads may or may not return to previous levels. If not, a sufficiently large fee increase would still allow physicians to earn the same income as previously.

In other instances, however, the physician's discretionary power may be more limited. Thus, in figure 2–5, demand is shifted out to D_3; physicians are able to increase visits from V_a to V_d, but not to raise fees as well. Price actually declines from P_a to P_d. Physicians' incomes (and possibly workloads as well) are likely to fall, but by a smaller amount than in the absence of an induced shift in demand. Empirically we cannot distinguish this new equilibrium price-quantity combination (D) from that observed at B. Lower prices and higher utilization rates are consistent with both the inducement and the neoclassical hypotheses.

How does inducement actually take place in the physician's or surgeon's practice? Faced with a declining caseload, the physician or surgeon may simply recommend (and perform) additional services for his or her remaining patients.[24] He or she chooses whether to recommend return office visits or more frequent checkups, for example, or whether to perform a certain medical or surgical procedure.

While surgeons may be able to reallocate some of their professional time into nonsurgical activities, their ability to do so will be constrained by the relative supply of other physician specialties. It is also reasonable to assume that surgeons will prefer to do surgery for two reasons. First, net hourly revenue will be higher for surgical activities, as the surgeon uses more free hospital inputs and incurs fewer office expenses. Second, the practice of surgery entails considerable professional prestige and personal satisfaction, which may be the reason why the surgeon chose this specialty.

Under conditions of high surgeon density, providers are hypothesized to exercise their discretionary ability to induce demand. They do so by encouraging surgical intervention for patients' conditions, when previously they might have recommended medical treatment. Given a high workload, surgeons are assumed to allocate time to nonelective surgical procedures. As they have more time available, however, they are apt to perform more elective procedures. For example, where before the surgeon might have advocated no treatment for silent gallstones, he or she now recommends a cholecystectomy. Rather than drug therapy for menstrual irregularities, a hysterectomy is now proposed.

The medical provider is hypothesized to shift demand in order to attain a target income. The target income is the amount of money earned through medical practice that the physician wants to achieve. The actual target is determined through comparison with other physicians of the same specialty training and geographic location.

Per-Capita Utilization

Recent studies of the impact of increases in the physician-population ratio on utilization are summarized in table 2-4. As shown, no studies report a fall in utilization associated with increases in physician supply. The empirical evidence indicates a modest positive relationship between utilization and

Table 2–4
Impact of Increase in Physician-Population Ratio on Services per Capita

Study	Type of Service	Elasticity
May 1975	Office visits	+.137
	Total visits	+.190
Fuchs 1978	Operations, 1970	+.236 to +.329
	Operations, 1963	+.232 to +.243
Holahan 1975	AFDC children	+.33[a]
	Disabled	+.39[a]
	AFDC adults	+.40[a]
Davis and Reynolds 1976	Elderly	+.80
Newhouse and Phelps 1976	Total sample	+.03
	Heads	+.17[a]
Fuchs and Kramer 1972	Physician visits	+.335 to +.507
Held and Manheim 1980	Expenditures	+.124
	Visits	+.077[a]

Source: Janet Mitchell and Jerry Cromwell, *Physician-Induced Demand for Surgical Operations* (Washington, D.C.: Health Care Financing Administration, Office of Research Demonstrations and Statistics, March 1981), p. 41.
a. Indicates the elasticity is not statistically significant.

the physician-population ratio. Estimated elasticities vary widely from 0.03 to 0.80 but appear to concentrate in the 0.24 to 0.40 range. In order to put these results in better perspective, several of the individual studies are discussed subsequently.

In their major study of physician services, Fuchs and Kramer estimated four structural equations: per-capita utilization, physician location, workload, and per-capita insurance benefits. The analysis was based on cross-section information that was collected in 1966 from 33 states. Per-capita utilization was expressed as a function of the net price of physician services, insurance benefits, physician supply, per-capita income, and the supply of hospital beds.

The predicted physician supply variable was positive and highly significant, with estimated elasticities ranging from +0.34 to +0.51. This implies that a 10 percent increase in the physician-population ratio will increase the quantity of visits demanded by 3 to 5 percent. Fuchs and Kramer note that this increase in utilization cannot be attributed to a fall in the money price of care, as average (or net) price was held constant in the demand equation. Given the low price elasticities in their equation (approximately −0.2), they also reject reductions in time price as a significant factor. However, as Sloan and Feldman have indicated, this is not necessarily true, if the time price constitutes a large proportion of total price.[25]

While most utilization studies have analyzed office visit rates, Fuchs examined the demand for surgical operations. Operations have several advantages as a measure of change in demand. In particular, reduced travel and waiting times are unlikely to lower the time price of surgery; the time price of hospitalization and psychic costs associated with the procedure (pain and suffering) are relatively more important.

Fuchs found a significant positive relationship between the supply of surgeons and the number of operations per capita in 1970, with elasticities ranging from +0.24 to +0.33 depending upon the equation specification. This implies that a 10 percent increase in the surgeon-population ratio results in 3 percent increase in the number of operations. Moreover differences in surgeon supply seem to have a perverse effect on physician fees, raising them when the surgeon-population ratio increases.[26]

Davis and Reynolds examined utilization rates for selected population groups: public-assistance recipients, other low-income persons, and the elderly.[27] Household self-reports from the 1969 Health Interview Survey formed the data base for their study. Physician-population ratios were calculated and merged with individual records in the following manner: by Standard Metropolitan Statistical Area (SMSA) for persons living in the twenty-two largest SMSAs, and by SMSA or non-SMSA residence within each of four census regions for all other persons. The latter specification is clearly inappropriate, and border crossing could produce substantial downard bias in regression coefficients.

The supply variable had a positive and significant relationship with physician vists for the elderly population, with a very high estimated elasticity of 0.80. Davis and Reynolds also found that the elasticity of physician utilization with respect to supply was substantially higher in urban than in rural areas, 0.81 compared with 0.54.

Omitted variables may have biased these elasticity estimates upward, however, as neither money nor time-price variables were included in these regressions. As physician-population ratios rise, lower physician fees and reduced travel and waiting times will increase the demand for visits, other things being equal.

Between 1969 and 1977 controlling for specialty and location, physicians' real incomes in the United States fell around 1.75 percent per year.[28] Moreover Canadian physicians' real incomes fell after various measures resulted in an increase in the number of Canadian physicians. If physicians have sufficient demand-creation ability to offset fully any adverse changes in the external environment, one presumes they would not tolerate a decline in real income. Thus even if the elasticity estimates presented are correct, the ability of providers to stimulate demand is limited.

Summary

Several important problems must be considered when undertaking empirical studies of the demand for health care. The first is the adequacy of using health-insurance information to obtain estimates of the price of health services. The second is the effect of provider influence on demand (the extent to which supply creates its own demand). The third problem is the effect on health status on the demand for health care. Exclusion of a health-status variable will bias the results.

Empirical studies indicate that health service demand is inelastic with respect to price and income. The elasticity of the time price of health care (the price of both waiting time and travel time) is low in an absolute sense but clearly important.

Most studies indicate that physicians and surgeons do create demand for their own services. However, the decline in physicians' incomes from 1969 to 1977 indicates that this demand-creation effect may be limited.

Notes

1. Richard Leftwich, *The Price System and Resource Allocation* (New York: Holt, Rinehart, and Winston, 1960), p. 27.

2. David Salkever and Alan Sorkin, "Economics, Health Economics, and Health Administration," report prepared for the Association of University Programs in Health Administration, August 1976 (mimeographed), p. 11.

3. Leftwich, *Price System and Resource Allocation*, p. 28.

4. Alfred Marshall, *Principles of Economics*, 8th ed. (London: MacMillan, 1920), book III, ch. 10.

5. Engel curves are named after Ernst Engel, a German pioneer of the last half of the nineteenth century in the field of budget studies. See George J. Stigler, "The Early History of Empirical Studies of Consumer Behavior," *Journal of Political Economy* 62, no. 2 (April 1954): 98–100.

6. The notion of time price is related to the concept of opportunity cost. Opportunity cost relates to foregone earning or consumption alternatives when one pursues a preferred course of action.

7. Michael Grossman, *The Demand for Health: A Theoretical and Empirical Investigation* (New York: Columbia University Press for the National Bureau of Economic Research, 1972).

8. Salkever and Sorkin, "Economics, Health Economics, and Health Administration," p. 36.

9. Hyman Joseph, "Empirical Research on the Demand for Health Care," *Inquiry* 8, no. 1, (March 1971): 62.

10. Salkever and Sorkin, "Economics, Health Economics, and Health Administration, p. 32.

11. Martin Feldstein, "Hospital Cost Inflation: A Study of Nonprofit Price Dynamics," *American Economic Review* 61, no. 5 (December 1971):

853–872; Karen Davis and R. Reynolds, "Medicare and the Utilization of Health Services by the Elderly," *Journal of Human Resources* 10, no. 3 (Summer 1975): 361; J. Holahan, "Physician Availability, Medical Care Reimbursement and Delivery of Physician Services: Some Evidence from the Medicaid Program," *Journal of Human Resources* 10, no. 3 (Summer 1975): 378.

12. If need were uncorrelated with other independent variables, its omission in a demand equation would not bias the statistical results.

13. Milton Friedman and Simon Kuznets, *Income from Independent Professional Practice* (New York: National Bureau of Economic Research, 1945), pp. 157–158.

14. Ronald Andersen, *A Behavioral Model of Families' Use of Health Services*, Center for Health Administration Studies, Research Series 25 (Chicago: Graduate School of Business, The University of Chicago, 1968).

15. Ibid., pp. 31 and 33.

16. Karen Davis and Louise Russell, "The Substitution of Hospital Outpatient Care for Inpatient Care," *Review of Economics and Statistics* 54, no. 2 (May 1972): 109–120; Paul Feldstein, *Financing Dental Care* (Lexington, Mass.: D.C. Heath, 1973).

17. A.G. Holtmann and E.R. Olsen, Jr., *The Economics of the Private Demand for Outpatient Health Care*, John E. Fogarty International Center for Advanced Studies in the Health Sciences, DHEW Publication no. (NIH) 78-1262 (Washington, D.C.: U.S. Government Printing Office, 1978), p. 75.

18. J. Acton, *Demand for Health Care among the Urban Poor with Special Emphasis on the Role of Time* (Santa Monica, Cal.: Rand, 1973), pp. 1–52.

19. Paul Feldstein, *Health Care Economics* (New York: John Wiley and Sons, 1979), p. 83.

20. Jacques Van Der Gaag and Mark Perlman (Eds.), *Health, Economics, and Health Economics*, Proceedings of the World Congress on Health Economics, Leiden, Netherlands, September 1980 (New York: North Holland, 1981), p. 95.

21. David Guzick, "Demand for General Practitioner and Internist Services," *Health Services Research* 13, no. 4 (Winter 1978): 351.

22. Grossman, *Demand for Health*.

23. Janet Mitchell and Jerry Cromwell, "Physician-Induced Demand for Surgical Operations" (Washington, D.C.: U.S. Department of Health and Human Services, Health Care Financing Administration, Office of Research, Demonstrations and Statistics. March 1981), p. 31.

24. Ibid., p. 91.

25. Frank Sloan and Roger Feldman, "Monopolistic Elements in the Market for Physicians' Services," in Warren Greenberg (Ed.), *Competition*

in the Health Care Sector: Past, Present, and Future, Proceedings of a conference sponsored by the Federal Trade Commission, March 1978, pp. 57–131.

26. Victor Fuchs, "The Supply of Surgeons and the Demand for Operations," *The Journal of Human Resources*, Vol. 13, Supplement, 1978, p. 35.

27. Karen Davis and Roger Reynolds, "The Impact of Medicare and Medicaid on Access to Medical Care," in Richard Rosett (Ed.), *The Role of Health Insurance in the Health Services Sector* (New York: National Bureau of Economic Research, 1976), pp. 391–425.

28. Van Der Gaag and Perlman, *Health, Economics, and Health Economics*, p. 94.

3   Health Manpower

A variety of economic issues are related to manpower in the health-care field. Consideration is given in this chapter to techniques of projecting the need for manpower, to the use of health auxiliaries in both rich and poor nations and to the severity of the shortage of physicians as well as other health personnel in the United States, the maldistribution of physicians, and the problems associated with the emigration of health professionals to the United States from developing countries.

The Supply and Demand for Health Personnel

Before considering a number of projections that have been made regarding demand and supply of health workers, it is important to understand the distinction between the terms *requirements* and *supplies* as used in various health manpower projections and the economists' concepts of supply and demand.

The terms *requirements* and *supplies* have rather special meanings. They refer to the quantity of labor services that will be demanded and supplied assuming that the relative structure of prices and earnings remains the same. Thus requirements and supplies are not the same as the economists' concepts of *demand* and *supply*, since the latter indicate the *schedules* of the quantities demanded and supplied at various prices. Requirements and supplies can be considered as being points on future demand and supply schedules at some previous year's price levels. Since the discussions that accompany projections often assume no possibility of demand and supply being equal at some price (a shortage exists), requirements and supplies can be portrayed respectively as vertical demand and supply schedules.[1]

The difference between these concepts is illustrated below. Figure 3–1 shows the traditional demand (D) and supply (S) schedules, relating quantities supplied and demanded at various prices. The fact that they intersect indicates the possibility of equilibrium in the market; at some price P_1 the quantity demanded will equal the quantity supplied. That equilibrium situation occurs at A. Generally it is assumed that as supply (S') and demand (D') shift in the future, some new price will result as indicated by P_2. In this case the greater relative increase in demand leads to a price increase, and the quantity supplied and demanded at price P_2 is indicated by A'.

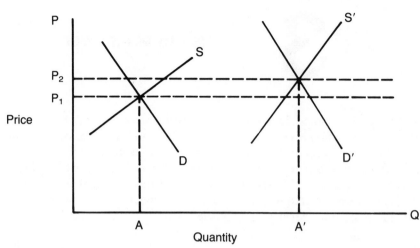

Source: Adapted from W. Lee Hansen, "An Appraisal of Physician Manpower Projections," *Inquiry* 7, no. 1 (March 1970: 103

Figure 3–1. Relationship of Demand (*D*) to Supply (*S*) at Various Price Levels (*P*)

The approach implied by projections of requirements and supply is indicated in figure 3–2. One starts from an initial position, quantity *A* and price P_1, which reflects the prevailing supply and demand conditions. Projected requirements *R* and projected supplies *SS* in some future year are shown as points, the quantities that will be supplied and demanded at price P_1. However, because there is a gap between *SS* and *R* of *MN*, and since the assumptions underlying most manpower projections preclude price changes that might alter the quantities supplied or demanded, this implies a set of perfectly inelastic supply (*S'*) and demand (*D'*) curves. The only solution possible when prices are ignored is to augment supply by shifting *S'* outward to the right or moving *D'* to the left, or by some combination of shifts so that *S'* and *D'* converge. If supply and demand curves of the usual type (as in figure 3–1) were assumed, however, a gap equal to *MN* at price P_1 would still exist and the price would simply rise to P_2, automatically eliminating the shortage.

A different mode of analysis is necessary to study the labor market for nurses. Most nurses are employed by hospitals or nursing homes, which exert a dominant force in the market. The labor market for nurses is thus monopsonistic or oligopsonistic.

An essential characteristic of both monopsony and oligopsony is that the individual firm faces an upward-sloping curve for labor services rather than

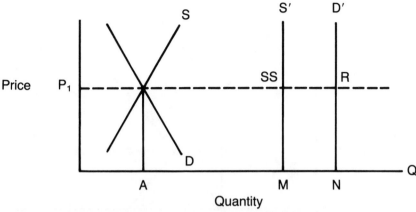

Source: Adapted from W. Lee Hansen, "An Appraisal of Physician Manpower Projections," *Inquiry* 7, no. 1 (March 1970): 103.

Figure 3–2. Relationship of Projected Requirements (R) to Projected Supply (SS) at a Fixed Price (P)

the horizontal supply curve faced by the firms in a perfectly competitive market. The consequences of this fact are that "If the supply curve to an individual firm is rising, the marginal cost of labor exceeds its average cost. An employer who is maximizing his profits will, therefore, offer no more although he may report vacancies."[2]

This situation is illustrated in figure 3–3, which shows a rising supply curve *S* and a corresponding marginal cost curve *MC* that is above *S* for all levels of employment. An employer faced with this situation will continue to hire more workers until the value of the marginal product is equal to the marginal cost (until the demand curve intersects the marginal cost curve). At this point the company will employ *ON* labor, pay a wage of *OW*, and report vacancies *NM*. The employer will not be willing to pay higher salaries but will be willing to hire more labor at the prevailing wage. Under these circumstances vacancies *cannot* reasonably be called excess demand and will not exercise any upward pressure on wages. Moreover in a monopsony situation an increase in demand relative to supply will cause wages to rise and reported vacancies to increase, so that assuming an imperfect market and an employer's goal of profit maximization, "a large number of reported vacancies may be perfectly consistent with equilibrium in the labor market."[3]

Part of the explanation for the chronic reports of unfilled nurse positions is the concentration of nurse employment in hospitals (which are hiring nurses on a monopsonistic basis). While the equilibrium vacancies reported by hospitals represent a misallocation of nursing resources, they do not result from market disequilibrium.

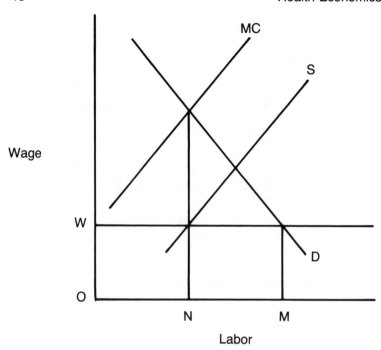

Figure 3–3. Model of a Monopsonistic Labor Market

This does not mean that throughout most of the postwar period there has been no shortage of nurses. It does mean, though, that reported vacancy rates do not accurately depict the magnitude of this shortage.

Methods of Determining Shortage

A variety of methods have been used to determine the magnitude of the physician shortage. The first is termed the *biologic demand* approach. In a study completed in 1933, Roger Lee and Lewis Jones estimated the *need* for physicians based on a consensus among experts regarding the amount of care—the number of physician hours—required to prevent, diagnose, and treat specific diseases and health conditions. The study translated the number of hours needed into a physician requirement based on the number of hours worked per year by each physician. The requirement was 134.7 physicians per 100,000 population (about 165,000 physicians for the nation). The 1930 census listed 154,000 active physicians.[4] Since not all of these physicians were available for full-time patient care, according to the criteria developed by Lee and Jones, these was a shortage of physicians.

The biological demand approach has a number of weaknesses. First, morbidity rates change, as do the number of hours required to treat a particular condition. Technological change in the health-care industry prevents this method from being accurate for long-term projections.

Second, the problem of health manpower is examined solely in terms of need. In a society in which goods and services are bought and sold in a market, this will overstate the demand for physicians because of financial, geographical, and other barriers to care. However, if demand were being projected for physicians in a society where there were no financial barriers to health care (such as the National Health Service in the United Kingdom), need and effective demand would be more similar. The biological demand approach would be appropriate.

A third weakness of the biological demand method is that it puts the whole emphasis on professional standards; that is, on what physicians think is necessary. Professional standards are in no sense absolutes. They do not replace the need for allocation decisions by those who must view the competing demands of the various sectors of society: health, education, water development, smog control, transportation, housing, or food. As long as resources are scarce, these allocation decisions will be required.

The biologic demand method was replicated about 40 years after the Lee–Jones report in a study by Schonfeld, Heston, and Falk. The latter estimated the number of physicians (pediatricians and internists) required for primary medical care. They found that primary medical care of good quality requires the services of 133 physicians per 100,000 persons of all ages in the population. Since the population at the time of the study was about 200 million, this meant about 266,000 physicians were needed for primary medical care. According to the authors there were only 59 primary-care physicians per 100,000 in 1970, indicating a severe shortage of primary-medical-care practitioners.[5]

A second method to be considered for estimating labor shortages is the manpower/population ratio. This approach either assumes that the present ratio of, for example, dentists to population is adequate or that an ideal dentist/population ratio can be specified. Future requirements are simply the expected future population times the present or ideal dentist/population ratio.

For example, if in a population of 300,000 persons there were 400 dentists, this would indicate a dentist/population ratio of 1 dentist per 750 persons. If this ratio were deemed appropriate and it was expected that in the next 10 years population would increase by 80 percent, the number of dentists would have to rise to 720 to maintain the dentist/population ratio.

The greatest advantage of this approach is the ease of calculation and the ready availability of data on the number of persons actively employed in various health occupations, as well as statistics on total population, for both developed and developing countries. However, there are a number of disadvantages to this method of determining requirements for health manpower.

The approach ignores changes in the composition of the population, thereby disregarding each population subgroup's characteristic demands for health services. For example, a shift in the population toward older age groups will increase health services demand by a faster rate than mere growth of total population.

A second disadvantage is that using, for example, the existing physician/population ratio to estimate future requirements for physicians assumes that the productivity increase of the present stock of physicians is zero. This is unrealistic, since studies have shown substantial and consistent increases in the productivity of physicians and dentists over time.[6] The more rapid the rate of increase in productivity, the smaller the increase in the number of health workers needed.

The final criticism of this approach is that it does not consider the substitution of other types of health workers for the type of personnel under consideration. For example, there will be a smaller increase in demand for physicians if some of their responsibilities are undertaken by physician's assistants. There will be a lessened demand for dentists if some of their responsibilities are carried out by dental hygienists.

One of the most frequent applications of the manpower/population method is the study of spatial or geographic maldistribution. The relative adequacy of manpower for different states, counties, or regions is frequently based on comparisons of manpower/population ratios.

Given the inadequacies of the foregoing approach, Rashi Fein developed a method for determining the change in demand for *health services* that would take into account the changing composition of the population. An analyst using Fein's method would project current physician utilization rates into the future, keeping them constant for each socioeconomic-demographic population subgroup. The total change in demand is attributed to both changes in the number as well as the composition of the population.

Aside from focusing attention on the effect of the changing composition of the population on the demand for health manpower, Fein shifted emphasis from the demand for health workers to the demand for health services.

> The first step in our analysis requires that we distinguish physician manpower from physician services and the latter from health, the ultimate goal. . . . The link between manpower and services is close but if our interest is in services and surely if it is in health, we cannot focus simply on manpower. Technology is changed, capital equipment is modified, and new organizations for the delivery of health services are created. All these may alter the relation between the "input" called the physician and the product he delivers . . . the health service . . . It should be remembered that a

patient's health is not improved by manpower itself but by the services it may provide.[7]

For Fein the unit of service was the physician visit. His results indicated that the demand for physician visits would increase between 22 and 26 percent between 1965 and 1975, and 35 to 40 percent by 1980.[8] About four-sevenths of the projected increase in demand between 1965 and 1975 was accounted for by growth of the total population. Thus about three-sevenths of the growth in demand is due to other quantifiable factors that would have been ignored in the more traditional physician/population ratio projections. Fein expected the supply of physicians would increase by 19 percent, or about 3 to 7 percent less than the demand for physicians' services. He expected that the shortage of physicians would worsen from 1965 to 1975.

It should be noted that Fein's approach does not indicate the magnitude of the physician shortage at any point in time. It does indicate whether, over time, an existing shortage is becoming more severe, less severe, or remaining the same. Moreover Fein's approach does not directly consider productivity or organizational changes within the health system and the effect of these on the overall magnitude of the shortage.

Fein's projections both of demand and supply of services were too low. His projections of demand did not adequately consider the effect of Medicare and Medicaid on health-services utilization. Since the forecasts were made while the programs were just being implemented, neither Fein nor anyone else could have foreseen the impact of these two programs on the demand for services. Fein's supply estimates were too low because he failed to anticipate the increase in the number of foreign medical graduate practicing in this country.

A fourth approach to the problem of manpower shortages is known as the *relative income method*. Using this criteria, there is evidence of a shortage in a particular occupation when salaries increase more rapidly over time than in *comparable occupations*. For example, from 1959 to 1969 the median earnings of physicians rose from $22,100 to $40,500, an increase of 87 percent.[9] In contrast, the increase for professional and technical workers was 61 percent.[10] The rate of increase for manufacturing workers for a comparable time period was only 43 percent. Using this criteria, the shortage of physicians worsened during the 1960s. However, from 1970 to 1979 physicians' incomes rose 88 percent, below the rate of increase for manufacturing workers (101 percent) but above the 75 percent gain for professional and technical workers. This would imply that during the 1970s the physician shortage did not become less severe.[11]

There are several objections to this method of identifying manpower shortages, an approach first utilized in an analysis of the shortage of engineers. First, the lag in adjustment to dynamic changes in demand is not considered and neither the beginning nor direction of the shortage is directly ascertainable. Moreover, a major problem is entailed in determining the choice of an appropriate or comparison group. For example, are all professional and technical workers an appropriate reference group for physicians? Finally, this approach does not consider the cost of training or changes in the cost of training over time. The income of a particular occupation may rise relative to others, but this may simply reflect higher training costs for the former occupation, with little change in net lifetime income.

An investment concept known as the *internal rate of return* considers both the cost of training and the economic returns that accrue to individuals who have obtained training. This amounts to considering training as an investment in human capital that yields a continuing flow of money returns.

According to this method, trends in rates of return to training in a particular occupation indicate what is happening with respect to the magnitude of the shortage. If rates of return are rising relative to those for comparable groups, the shortage is becoming more severe. If the rates of return are declining relative to that of an appropriate reference group, the shortage is becoming less severe. This concept of shortage can be illustrated with respect to dentists. (See table 3–1.)

Although the estimates of return differ significantly because of methodological variations in the calculations, there is no evidence that the shortage of dentists became more severe from 1939 to 1958. Maurizi and Feldstein's

Table 3–1
Rates of Return to Dental Education, 1939–1970

Year	Hansen	Maurizi	Feldstein
1939	12.3		
1948		19.1	
1949	13.4		
1952		21.0	
1955		18.5	
1956	12.0		
1958		14.8	
1960			17.5
1961		17.9	
1965			24.2
1970		25.5	24.5

Source: W. Lee Hansen, "Shortages and Investment in Health Manpower," in *The Economics of Health and Medical Care*, Proceedings of the Conference and the Economics of Medical Care, May 10–12, 1962 (Ann Arbor: University of Michigan, School of Public Health, 1964), p. 86; Alex Maurizi, "Rates of Return in the Dental Profession," *Economic Essays on the Dental Profession* (Iowa City: University of Iowa, 1969), p. 13; Paul Feldstein, *Financing Dental Care: An Economic Analysis* (Lexington, Mass.: Lexington Books, D.C. Heath, 1973), p. 91; and Alex Maurizi, "Rates of Return to Dentistry and the Decision to Enter Dental School," *Journal of Human Resources* 10, no. 4 (Fall 1975): 524.

data do indicate that the shortage of dentists worsened during the 1960s as the rates of return to dentistry rose significantly.

The major difficulty with using trends in rates of return to study changing degrees of labor shortages is that such an analysis assumes a highly competitive labor market. However, the health-care industry is not a competitive one and there are major monopolistic or oligopolistic elements in the labor market for physicians, dentists, or veterinarians. Thus an increase in the rate of return to medical education could occur, for example, if the American Medcial Association were to gain greater control over some segment of the medical-care market and not because of any increase in the shortage of physicians. However, during the 1960s the influence of the AMA may have declined (since a declining proportion of physicians were members of the association) and the rates of return to medical education rose sharply. Thus it is highly likely that this reflected a genuine shortage situation.

A final approach to determining the magnitude of future shortages, reflecting the future demand and supply of health manpower is by using econometric models. These models, some of which have dozens of variables, use computers to calculate the results.

For example, one relatively simple model considered the supply and demand for allied health personnel.[12]

The demand equation was

$$PAR^D = f \left(PD_H, PD_{NH}, OPV, DOV, HC, W_{PAR}, \frac{W_{PAR}}{W_N}, \frac{W_{MD_p})}{W_{PAR}} \right.$$

The supply equation was

$$PAR^S = f \; \frac{(W_{PAR}}{W_R}, \frac{W_{PAR})}{CPI}$$

where

PAR_D = number of employed paramedical personnel per thousand population;

PD_H = hospital patient days per thousand population;

OPV = number of out-patient visits per thousand population;

DOV = number of doctor's office visits per thousand population per year;

HC = days of home care received per thousand population;

$\dfrac{W_{PAR}}{W_N}$ = $\dfrac{\text{wages of paramedics}}{\text{wage of nurses}}$

$$\frac{W_{MD_P}}{W_{PAR}} = \frac{\text{wages of physicians}}{\text{wages of paramedics}}$$

W_R = weekly income in retail trade

$$\frac{W_{PAR}}{CPI} = \frac{\text{wage of paramedics}}{\text{consumer price index}}$$

The Graduate Medical Education National Advisory Committee (GMENAC) developed models for projection of the supply and demand for physicians from 1978 to 2000. These estimates were made not only for physician manpower as a whole, but for a number of medical specialties.[13]

The supply model projects for a future year the number of physicians in the aggregate or in each specialty. The model considers present supply, the number of U.S. medical school graduates, foreign medical graduates (FMGs), and residents in training, and the proportion changing specialties during graduate medical education or later, and finally it adjusts for death, disability, and retirement.

The requirements model is a hybrid between need-based and demand-based methods. The model takes into account both demand-based data, which reflects current utilization patterns, and need-based figures based on the provision of all services needed by the entire population. The model adjusts those latter figures based on what can realistically be accomplished. The adjustments are partly based on a Delphi Panel of six to ten experts for each specialty.

Using these models, GMENAC has projected a surplus of physicians in 1990 with substantial imbalances in a number of specialties. The panel indicated a shortage of physicians in 1978 but projected a growing surplus in the future:[14]

Year	Demand	Supply
1978	419,000	375,000
1990	466,000	536,000
2000	498,000	643,000

The ratio of physicians to population, which was 171 per 100,000 in 1978, is projected to jump to 220 per 100,000 in 1990, and 247 per 100,000 in 2000.

Although the projections indicated a substantial overall surplus of physicians by 1990, a number of specialties were still expected to exhibit shortages. (See table 3–2.)

In order to minimize the expected surplus, the panel recommended three significant actions:

1. Reduce enrollments in American Medical schools by 10–15 percent. At present there are approximately 70,000 students in the nation's medical schools.
2. Restrict greatly the number of graduates of foreign medical schools who are permitted to practice medicine in the United States. The 40,000 to 50,000 foreign graduates expected to begin practice here in the 1980s account for the bulk of the projected surplus.
3. In view of the aggregate surplus of physicians projected for 1990, medical school graduates in the 1980s should be strongly encouraged to enter those specialties where a shortage of physicians is expected (see table 3–2), or to enter training and practice in general pediatrics, general internal medicine, and family practice.

The panel recommended that to encourage students to become primary-care physicians rather than surgical specialists, the early phase of medical school should emphasize "a broad-based clinical experience" and put "a more vigorous and imaginative emphasis . . . on ambulatory care."

Health Manpower Legislation

From the early 1960s until the mid 1970s there was a basic presumption that a shortage of health professionals existed. Therefore the legislation was increasingly in the direction of encouraging health professions' schools to expand. Since 1976 it has been generally recognized that shortages of

Table 3–2
Supply and Requirements, Selected Specialties, 1990

Specialty	Supply	Requirements	Surplus (Shortage)
General psychiatry	30,500	38,500	(8,000)
Emergency medicine	9,250	13,500	(4,250)
Preventive medicine	5,650	7,300	(1,750)
Dermatology	7,350	6,950	400
Family practice	58,200	61,300	(3,100)
Urology	6,050	7,700	(1,650)
Ophthalmology	6,900	11,600	(4,700)
Plastic Surgery	3,900	2,700	1,200
General Surgery	35,300	23,500	11,800
Neurosurgery	5,100	2,650	2,450
Obstetrics/gynecology	34,450	24,000	10,450
General pediatrics and subspecialties	41,350	36,400	4,950

Source: U.S. Department of Health and Human Services, *Summary Report of the Graduate Medical Education National Advisory Committee*, DHHS Publication no. (HRA)81-651 (Washington, D.C.: U.S. Government Printing Office, 1980), p. 5.

various categories of health professionals no longer exist and that surpluses are expected, as in the case of physicians, for example. In response to this changing situation, health labor legislation has become increasingly restrictive.

The passage of the Health Professions Education Assistance Act of 1963 marked a major shift in federal policy. This law provided, for the first time, funds for school construction and student loans.[15] Thus $175 million was authorized for matching grants for construction to be given to schools training individuals for health careers at the professional level. The act permitted the grants to cover up to two-thirds of the cost of construction or major expansion.[16]

Several important additions and modifications to federal programs supporting manpower training were included in the Health Manpower Act of 1968. The law provided for increased federal matching funds in cases where a medical or nursing school was experiencing financial difficulties resulting from large expenses for projects such as major revisions in curriculum, replacement of obsolete facilities, or moving to a new location. Moreover greater federal support was extended to schools of nursing, pharmacy, and veterinary medicine.

The student loan program was expanded. The funds available were increased from $25 million to $35 million, but a reduction was made in the grace period for repaying loans except for students receiving advanced professional training.[17]

The Comprehensive Health Manpower Training Act of 1971, in effect during the years 1972–1976, was a major piece of health-manpower training legislation. It provided for four major types of financial assistance: construction support, institutional aid, student loans and scholarships, and funding for special programs.

The 1971 law authorized three kinds of construction assistance: grants, interest subsidies, and loan guarantees. It raised the grant allowable for any project to 70 percent of the total cost, except for expansion programs, in which case grants of 80 percent of cost could be obtained.

The act also provided basic institutional support in the form of capitation payments.[18] To qualify for a capitation grant, each school was required to increase its first year enrollment by a specified percentage.

A participating institution received a basic amount for each student, a higher amount for each graduate, and a bonus for students in classes that exceed the required increased enrollment by 5 percent or five students, whichever was larger.

The federal government provided two kinds of assistance to health professions' students. The help was composed of loans and scholarships. To receive loan funds under the 1971 act, the school was required to contribute $1 from its own funds for every $9 contributed by the federal government. No loan could exceed $3,500 per year, and the interest rate charged the student could not exceed 3 percent.

The 1971 act also included generous loan-forgiveness provisions. The government could forgive or repay 85 percent of any outstanding loan for a student who agreed to practice for 3 years in an area with a health-manpower shortage. There was also provision for the repayment of loans for students from low-income families who did not complete their professional training.

Health-Professions Assistance Act of 1976

In October 1976 President Ford signed HRS 546, a major piece of health manpower legislation. This law, which was not significantly changed from 1976 to 1980, reflected a belief in government that there was no longer a shortage of most categories of health professionals. The major provisions of the bill were as follows:[19]

1. The federal loan program was replaced by a program of federal loan guarantees. The maximum annual loan a student could receive was $10,000, with a limitation of total indebtedness of $50,000. The government canceled $10,000 of the loan for each year a student agreed to practice in a location with a shortage of health personnel.
2. A small direct-loan program was maintained, but only exceptionally needy students were eligible in 1979–80. The law increased the maximum annual loan from $2,500 to $3,500 but also increased the interest rate from 3 to 7 percent.
3. The federal scholarship program was extensively changed. A general program of scholarship support was discontinued. Nearly all scholarships were reserved for persons who join the National Health Service Corps and thus were serving in federally designated shortage areas.
4. Each school of medicine, osteopathy, and dentistry received $2,000 in capitation grants in 1978 and $2,100 in 1980. Schools were required to maintain first-year enrollment levels in the following fiscal year and maintain the level of nonfederal expenditures realized the previous year.
5. The 1976 law eliminated immigration preferences for alien graduates of foreign medical schools who had not passed medical qualifying examinations and demonstrated competency in written and oral English. In addition, regulations were developed making it more difficult for foreign medical graduates to obtain exchange visitor visas.

    Because may hospitals depend on foreign medical graduates for house staff positions, the new requirements for exchange visitor visas were waived until December 31, 1980. This delay gave hospitals time to develop alternative manpower sources.

6. Federal support for the construction of medical facilties was cut drasti-
    cally to $40 million annually from 1978 to 1980. This reflected the
    position that the country no longer needed to increase the overall supply
    of health manpower.

Table 3–3 summarizes the authorizations from 1976 to 1980 under the
Health Professions Education Assistance Act of 1976. From 1976 to 1980
changes in health-manpower legislation were very minor. Public Law 96-76,
passed in September 1979, increased the level of student loans for those
studying medicine, dentistry, and osteopathy from $10,000 to $15,000 per
year, and from $50,000 to $60,000 in the aggregate.[20] Moreover the service
obligation of those participating in the National Health Service Corps could
be deferred up to 3 years to obtain further training. The legislation also

Table 3–3

**Summary of PL 94-484 Authorizations for Health Professions Education
($ millions)**

	Fiscal Year 1977	Fiscal Year 1978	Fiscal Year 1979	Fiscal Year 1980
Construction	127.0	42.0	43.0	43.0
Institutional support				
Capitation	133.7	——	——	——
Medicine		124.2	131.7	139.4
Osteopathy		8.7	9.3	10.2
Dentistry		43.8	45.4	46.9
Capitation	29.3	——	——	——
Veterinary medicine	——	10.2	10.6	10.7
Optometry	——	3.2	3.3	3.4
Pharmacy	——	17.0	17.1	17.4
Podiatry	——	2.3	2.3	2.3
Capitation—public health	——	9.7	10.5	11.1
Student assistance				
Student Loans	39.1	26.0	27.0	28.0
National Health Service Corps				
scholarships	40.0	75.0	140.0	200.0
Scholarships for exceptionally				
needy	——	16.0	17.0	18.0
Special Projects				
Family medicine training	39.0	45.0	45.0	50.0
Area health education centers	——	20.0	30.0	40.0
General internal medicine and				
general pediatrics	10.0	15.0	20.0	25.0
Occupational health training				
centers	5.0	5.0	8.0	10.0

Source: U.S. Department of Health and Human Services, Public Health Service, *Chronology:
Health Professions Legislation, 1956–1979*, DHHS Publication no. (HRA)80-69 (Washington,
D.C.: Department of Health and Human Services, August 1980), pp. 62–63.

extended much of the legislation concerning nursing scholarships and loans through 1983. In 1980, $101 million was appropriated for nurse trianing programs

The Omnibus Budget Reconciliation Act of 1981

The Omnibus Budget Reconciliation Act of 1981 detailed major cuts in federal expenditures in many sectors. Federal health manpower expenditures were cut substantially. Thus capitation grants to schools of medicine, osteopathy, dentistry, and veterinary medicine were eliminated.[21] Only schools of public health will be able to receive funding under this program for the fiscal years 1982–1984.

Funding for National Health Service Corps scholarships is 40 percent lower in 1982–1984 than in 1980. The student loan program is continued, but funding in 1982 was 25 percent below 1980. Moreover the Omnibus bill sharply reduced the funding for scholarships for the exceptionally needy, with funding 60 percent less in 1982–1984 than in 1980.

This law provided no additional funding for construction expenditures on behalf of schools of medicine, osteopathy, dentistry, or veterinary medicine. It did permit the secretary to make all authorized interest subsidy payment on any loan made under these programs prior to October 1, 1981, however, and provided $4.3 million for fiscal years 1982, 1983, and 1984 to meet these outstanding obligations.[22]

One likely effect of these budget cuts is that it will be more difficult for young people from low- to moderate-income families to choose a career in one of the health professions.

Table 3–4 indicates trends in enrollment and growth rates for selected health professions. A comparison is made between rates of growth in 1955–1966 (before the initiation of major federal programs) and 1966–1976 (when the programs were expanding).

These annual rates of increase strongly suggest that the various federal programs described have had a very substantial effect on enrollment and graduates. In nearly every case the percentage increase is several times higher in 1966–1976 as compared to 1955–1966.

The Distribution of Physicians

In 1923 89 percent of all physicians in the United States were general practitioners.[23] By 1976 this figure had fallen to 16 percent. The decline in the general practitioner had in many areas reduced access to primary health

Table 3-4
Number of Students Enrolled and Graduated 1955-56, 1965-66, and 1975-76; and Annual Rates of Increase 1956-66 and 1966-1976

	Students Enrolled			Percentage Increase	
	1955-1956	1965-1966	1975-1976	1956-1966	1966-1976
Physicians	30,522	34,516	56,244	13.1	63.0
Dentists	12,730	14,020	29,767	13.3	48.1
Registered nurses	102,853	135,702	213,127[a]	31.9	57.1[c]
Optometrists	1,233	1,745	3,931	41.5	125.2
Pharmacists	12,273	12,352	24,416	0.6	97.7
Podiatrists	700	694	2,085	-0.0	200.4
Veterinarians	3,419	4,119	6,400[b]	20.5	55.4
	Graduates			Percentage Increase	
	1955-1956	1965-1966	1975-1976	1956-1966	1966-1976
Physicians	7,309	7,934	13,561	8.6	70.9
Dentists	3,038	3,198	5,336	5.3	66.9
Registered nurses	28,539	35,125	58,300[a]	23.1	66.0[c]
Optometrists	333	384	905	15.3	135.7
Pharmacists	3,686	3,659	7,757	-0.7	112.0
Podiatrists	142	136	496	-4.2	264.7
Veterinarians	817	910	1,591	11.4	74.8

Source: Alan Sorkin, *Health Manpower: An Economic Perspective* (Lexington, Mass.: Lexington Books, D.C. Heath, 1977), p. 100; U.S. Department of Health, Education, and Welfare, *A Report to the President and Congress on the Status of Health Professions Personnel in the United States*, DHEW Publication no. (HRA)80-53 (Washington, D.C.: U.S. Government Printing Office, 1980), appendix, pp. A-1 to A-26.

a. Data for 1972-73.

b. Estimated.

c. Percentage increase 1966-1973.

care. General practitioners were the foundation of medical care in small and rural communities throughout the United States. As they died or retired, they were not being replaced by newly trained physicians.

As of 1978 the yearly production of family practitioners was still lower than the annual loss of general practitioners.[24] Furthermore it has been shown that retiring general practitioners are considerably more productive than the primary-care physicians who are now entering practice. The number of patients seen per hour and the number of hours worked per week are substantially lower for primary-care physicians now beginning practice than they are for retiring general practitioners.

Physicians are disproportionately located in the Northeast and the western region of the nation. The physician/population ratios in those areas are significantly higher than those in the south and north central states. For every 100,000 persons in South Dakota only 76 physicians provide patient care—a 1:1,316 ratio. This is contrasted with the figure of 195 physicians per 100,000 population in New York State, or a 1:500 ratio.[25]

Because the physician supply in nonmetropolitan and metropolitan areas grew at about the same rate during the 1970s, the gap in terms of the physician/population ratio between the two types of areas remained unchanged during the decade (at a ratio of about 2.3:1).[26]

However, the 35 percent growth rate in nonmetropolitan areas represented a significant improvement over the past situation. (See table 3–5.) Physician supply had grown only 11 percent during the 1960s—at less than one-third the rate of metropolitan counties. The change in the 1970s was greatest in the most isolated rural areas. While physician supply dropped 11 percent during the 1960s, between 1974 and 1978 it rose 23 percent— actually more than the national rate.

There are some important differences in the urban-rural distributions of various types of physicians. As table 3–6 indicates, general practitioners are quite evenly distributed, as are general surgeons. But there is a greater concentration of internists and pediatricians in urban areas, and a still

Table 3–5
Number and Percentage Change in Supply of Active MDs for Different Types of Areas, Selected Years, 1960–1978.

	Number			
	1960[a]	*1970*	*1974*	*1978*
U.S. Total	205,935	278,855	321,089	377,492
All metropolitan	170,792	239,831	276,97	324,627
Large metro core	94,303	129,125	143,286	160,707
Large metro fringe	16,209	28,301	35,309	44,115
Medium metro	43,941	60,526	72,817	88,108
Small metro	16,610	21,879	25,585	31,697
All nonmetropolitan	35,172	39,024	44,092	52,865
Isolated semirural	18,032	20,787	23,747	28,843
Isolated rural	2,507	2,219	2,416	2,975

	Percentage Change			
	1960–1970	*1970–1978*	*1970–1974*	*1974–1978*
U.S. total	+35	+35	+15	+18
All metropolitan	+40	+35	+15	+17
Large metro core	+37	+24	+11	+12
Large metro fringe	+75	+56	+25	+25
Medium metro	+38	+34	+20	+21
Small metro	+31	+45	+17	+24
All nonmetropolitan	+11	+35	+13	+20
Isolated semirural	+15	+39	+14	+21
Isolated rural	−11	+34	+ 9	+23

Source: U.S. Department of Health and Human Services, *Third Report to the President and Congress on the Status of Health Professions Personnel in the United States*, DHHS Publication no. (HRA)82-2 (Washington, D.C.: U.S. Department of Health and Human Services, January 1982), p. iv–96.

Table 3–6

A Comparison of the Urban-Rural Ratio of Physicians by Specialty

Specialty	Urban-Rural Ratio[a]
General family practice	0.7
General surgery	1.9
Obstetrics and gynecology	3.5
Pediatrics	4.0
Internal medicine	4.8
Thoracic surgery	5.5
Anesthesia	5.7
Psychiatry and Neurology	7.3
Neurosurgery	9.8

Source: American College of Surgeons and American Surgical Association, "Surgery in the United States: A Summary Report of the Study on Surgical Services for the United States," 1975; and G.A. Roback, "Distribution of Physicians in the United States, 1973," Center for Health Services and Research and Development (Chicago: American Medical Association, 1974). p.14.

a. Computed by dividing the number of urban-based physicians per capita by the number of rural-based physicians per capita.

greater concentration of non–primary-care specialists (except for general surgeons).

However, these is evidence that the number of specialists in nonurban areas is increasing. Although the extent of diffusion depended upon specialty, by 1977 it was common for communities of over 20,000 people to have board-certified specialists. The number of board-certified specialists in communities of 5,000 or more was typically two to four times greater in 1977 than in 1960.[27]

Allied Health Manpower

The federal government defines the term *allied health professions* as follows:

> Allied health manpower, when used broadly, covers all those professional, technical and supportive workers in the fields of patient care, community health, public health, environmental health, and health-related research who engage in activity that supports, complements or supplements the professional function of administrators, physicians and dentists.[28]

The total number of allied health workers rose from 1.5 to 2.6 million from 1960 to 1970, and from 2.6 to 3.5 million from 1970 to 1978.[29] These figures are all just estimates, because comprehensive data by allied health occupation do not exist.

In 1976, only about 1 million of over 3 million allied health personnel were employed in hospitals. Nursing-related services (mostly nurses' aides and orderlies) constitute two-fifths of all allied health personnel employed in hospitals, followed by administrative and clerical services (13 percent), clinical laboratory services (11 percent), and mental health and radiologic services (5 percent).[30]

During 1970–1975 allied health personnel constituted two-thirds of the staff in health-maintenance organizations, over three-fourths of nonphysician employees in physicians' offices, over two-thirds of employees in mental-health facilities, over three-fifths of the staffs in nursing and rest homes, and about one-fifth of the workers in college infirmaries.[31]

Because of the shortage of primary-care physicians and their geographic maldistribution, two new categories of midlevel health professionals began to be trained in the 1970s. These were the physician's assistants and the pediatric nurse practitioners.

According to DHEW estimates in 1980, there were aproximately 13,000 nurse practitioners in the United States and approximately 11,000 physician's assistants.[32] These two groups of midlevel health professionals are in some ways quite similar and in many other respects quite different.

In the United States the concept of the physician's assistant originated with the armed forces medical services. It was demonstrated that in 1 or 2 years it was possible to train young people with limited formal education to become skilled medical aides who screen patients, administer care, and perform intravenous transfusions and other technical procedures and tasks. To increase the supply of medical services, the concept has been transferred to the civilian community through physician's assistant training programs.

In 1970 the American Medical Association's Council on Health Manpower recommended to the AMA board of trustees the following working definition of the title *physician's assistant*:

> The physician's assistant is a skilled person qualified by academic training to provide patient services under the supervision and direction of a licensed physician who is responsible for the performance of that assistant.[33]

Researchers have developed a variety of methodologies to assess the productivity of physician's assistants. Scheffler, using a sample of 1,403 physician's assistants concluded that the average physician's assistant provided services equivalent to 0.63 physicians.[34]

In another study comparing practice settings with and without physician's assistants, it was observed that physician's assistants saw 79 percent as many patients as physicians. These figures are for a relatively small sample of 92 practices, however, and may not be representative of practices throughout the United States employing physician's assistants. (See table 3–7).

Table 3-7
An Estimate of the Productivity of Physician's Assistants

| | *Average Number of Patients Seen Weekly in Practice Setting by Individual Provider* | | | |
Type of Practice	Physician's Assistant	Supervising MD	Total Number of Patients Seen	MD in Comparable Practice Setting without PA
Solo practice	126	191	317	117
Nonpractice	95	107	202	146
Both practices combined (average for both)	104	132	236	139

Source: System Sciences, Inc., *Survey and Evaluation of Physician Extender Reimbursement Program*, Department of Health Education, and Welfare, Contract no. SSA-600-76-0167, Bethesda, Md, March 1978, pp. 48 and 51.

The productivity of physician's assistants who completed the Medex program indicated that during the year following Medex employment, the average number of office visits rose 12 percent, but 2 years later the average number had increased by 37 percent above the baseline level.[35] The average number of patient visits per day by supervising physicians remained essentially the same and the physician's assistant saw approximately half as many patients as the supervising physician. About 30 percent of the patients treated by a physician's assistant were also seen by the supervising physician.

The possibility exists that physicians might reduce their own patient load after employing a physician's assistant or nurse practitioner in order to have more leisure time or because they were previously overworked. If this occurs, the productivity gains attributed to physician's assistants would be limited.

In a study by the U.S. Comptroller General, 266 physicians supervising either physician's assistants or nurse practitioners were surveyed regarding working hours. Seventy percent reported no change in their working hours, 25 percent reported working fewer hours, and 5 percent reported working more hours after employing the physician's assistant.[36] In another survey physicians employing either physician's assistants or nurse practitioners ranked "increasing time for leisure," eleventh of thirteen consequences of the physician extender's employment upon the practice.[37]

Only one study is available which considered the profitability of physician's assistants. This study estimated the financial benefits of employing a physician assistant in twelve rural private practices. Each assistant had been employed for between 1 and 2 years. The researchers found the average physician's assistant's salary was $10,100, and an estimated increased overhead ranging from $5,900 to $10,000. Estimates of average revenues generated by each physician's assistant were between $28,190 and $30,210. On the basis of these computations, the profitability of employing an extender in these practices ranges between $8,100 and $14,300 annually.[38]

One of the important issues affecting the profitability of physician's assistants for their employers is the availability and rate of third-party reimbursement. The reluctance of Medicare and Medicaid to develop appropriate policies for reimbursing physicians who use nurse practitioners and physician's assistants is one of the factors impeding the utilization of these personnel. Institutions are permitted to apply the cost of employment of new health practitioners to Medicare A (hospital charges) or Medicaid. Private practices have not been able to pass these expenses on to third-party payers quite so readily.[39]

The development of the nurse-practitioner profession began in the early 1970s in response to: (1) nursing's opposition to the growth and development of physician's assistant training programs, (2) the increasing acceptance by patients of the concept of using nonphysicians in the diagnosis and treatment of common medical conditions, (3) growing recognition of a need for additional primary-care personnel, and (4) awareness of the need for challenging professional opportunities within the nursing profession.

Most nurse practitioners are one of three general types: (1) family nurse practitioner, (2) adult nurse practitioner, or (3) pediatric nurse practitioner. Training programs are either certificate programs, which do not confer a formal academic degree, or master's degree programs. The former usually last 4 to 6 months and train registered nurses. The master's degree programs are generally 1 year long and are limited to graduates of baccalaureate nursing programs. Most nurse-practitioner programs are administered by nurses, but they utilize physicians for clinical teaching and preceptorship. In almost all cases nurse-practitioner training programs are controlled by the nursing profession; and they appear to be using physicians less and less for teaching, particularly in master's programs.

According to Perry and Breitner, there will be almost 50 percent more nurse practitioners than physician's assistants by 1990.[40] However, if a larger number of nurse practitioners become professionally inactive after 5–10 years of employment, the number of employed physician's assistants may remain comparable to the number of employed nurse practitioners.

According to a study funded by the Department of Health, Education, and Welfare, nurse practitioners saw an average of 68 patients per week, whereas physician assistants saw 104.[41] Nurse practitioners generally saw between 5 and 14 patients per day, whereas almost all physician assistants saw more than 20 patients per day.

There may be several explanations for these findings. First, physician assistants are more likely to be working in fee-for-service private-practice settings than are nurse practitioners. The former encourage a rapid patient turnover.

Second, it is likely that part of the physician's assistant's greater productivity as compared to nurse practitioners arises form the former's greater involvement in the management of acute, self-limited conditions. It is possible that nurse practitioners are more likely to see patients with complex, multiple chronic problems.

Finally, physician's assistants work longer hours per week partly because of their concentration in fee-for-service settings (especially in rural areas), where night calls and longer workdays are required. Clinics, where nurse practitioners are concentrated, maintain much more restricted hours of operation.[42]

There is some concern that the expected surplus of physicians will reduce the demand for physician extenders. With a large increase in physicians, patient loads will tend to decline and physicians would be less likely to hire physician assistants. However, since nurse practitioners and physician's assistants tend to locate in areas short in health manpower, these professions may continue to expand. Moreover health-service system efficiency would increase and costs would likely rise more slowly if more medical services of a less complex nature were provided by personnel with less specialized training.

Medical Auxiliaries in Developing Countries

Several definitions of *auxiliary worker* exist. Roemer, in an analysis of the role of allied health personnel in developing and socialist countries, distinguishes four basic types of allied health workers: traditional healers, paramedical health workers, elementary doctor substitutes, and primary health practitioners.[43] In his scheme the paramedical health workers function under the strict supervision of doctors, carrying out specifically delegated functions. In this category is placed the nurse, except for the Latin American auxiliary nurse, who in practice takes the place of a physician in many rural areas. The elementary doctor substitute has a relatively broad role, and due to the lack of physicians in rural areas of developing countries, usually provides the bulk of the care for rural populations. The fourth category of health worker, the primary health practitioner, is known by a variety of terms: in the USSR *feldsher*, in Ethiopia *health officer*, and Malaysia *hospital assistant*.

Auxiliary health workers have also been classified by income and education levels as well as type of practice. In 1972 the World Health Organization defined the *medical assistant* as a health worker with eight to nine years basic general education followed by two or three years technical training that should enable him to recognize the most common diseases, to care for the simpler ones, to refer more complicated problems and cases to the nearest health center or hospital, to carry out preventive measures, and to promote health in his district.[44]

Most community health workers have less than 6 years of basic education and usually less than 1 year of professional training. They may undertake a broad range of activities, however, including personal and environmental health services and community-development tasks.

In terms of income, the auxiliary dresser, nurse's aide, auxiliary midwive, dispenser, and home health aide receive lower wages than the assitant medical officer, health officer, nurse, midwife, health visitor, and sanitarian. These in turn are less well paid than physicians, dentists, or sanitary engineers.[45]

The desire to extend service coverage into the village at low cost through the use of auxiliaries has been given additional impetus by the rapid rise in fuel costs. Areas that once relied on mobile medical teams now find these completely impractical. Increasing costs of medical care and manpower training further jeopardize adequate coverage of underserved areas.[46]

Nigeria, India, and Guatemala have developed reasonably effective low-cost village health programs. These programs use paraprofessionals who have been trained in maternal and child care, nutrition, and treatment of common medical problems. As a result major reductions have occurred in the mortality rates for infants and children 1 to 4 years old (in the sample populations). The cost per capita per year ranges from less than U.S.$0.50 to $2.00.

In an unusually detailed monograph on the structure, function, and evaluation of the Kavor (Iran) village health-care delivery system covering a rural population of 43,000, Ronaghy reported a cost per person of $3.50 and a cost of $2.55 per visit. In China, where financing of health care is local, it is estimated that the median cost per year (out-of-pocket) of the family membership premium is $5.00.[47]

One important argument in favor of auxiliaries is that many developing countries lack sufficient funds to train adequate numbers of physicians. Auxiliaries can be trained in far less time and at much lower cost. There is also a belief that auxiliary training can be better adapted to local educational attainment levels and the community's health needs, in terms of the most prevalent diseases in the locality. Village health auxiliaries are regarded by some as being better suited than physicians to provide health education, to record vital statistics, or to implement environmental sanitation programs in the community. They are assumed to know their communities well and to be culturally closer to the people they serve. Auxiliaries are also not likely to migrate to urban areas or to emigrate to more developed countries.

However, there are several arguments against the training and utilization of auxiliaries in developing countries. A major question is whether health duties can safely be delegated to them. Some fear more the possible mistakes of an ill-trained and poorly supervised auxiliary than they do the ills that afflict the people receiving no services at all.[48] Another issue is whether or not scarce economic resources should be diverted from medical education to auxiliary training. Some fear that the development of village health workers will retard the provision of higher-quality care by physicians. Also of concern is the possibility that auxiliaries will tend to become dissatisfied with their careers; that in fact they really wish to be physicians and will be discontent with a lesser status or will use auxiliary training as preparation for a career in politics. For these reasons some believe the auxiliary will lack commitment to the work, thus causing a high turnover of personnel and necessitating constant training programs. A further concern is that auxiliaries might set up their own practices—short-term practical health training may result in the auxiliary claiming to be far more knowledgeable than is really the case. Finally, many political leaders in developing countries consider auxiliary training institutions a relic of the colonial past. In the colonial period natives were frequently unable to be trained as health professionals in their own country. After independence reliance on training auxiliaries to provide the bulk of primary health care is often politically unacceptable.

Allied health workers make a major contribution to health care in developing countries. (See table 3–8.) Thus in many of the developing nations, the number of medical assistants is greater than the number of physicians and the number of assistant nurses exceeds the number of nurses.

Worldwide Trends in the Distribution of Health Manpower

Around 1975 the number of physicians per 100,000 inhabitants ranged between 140 and 180 or more for the developed regions. Among the developing regions, temperate South America also reached this level, with 158 physicians per 100,000 people. At the same time East Asia had 100 physicians to every 100,000 inhabitants; but the other developing regions lagged well behind, with not more than 65 physicians per 100,000 inhabitants. The regions least well-endowed with physicians are Middle Africa, West Africa, and East Africa, where there are not more than 6 physicians per 100,000 inhabitants. In other words proportionately to population, these three regions have 28 times fewer physicians than the more developed areas. Eastern South Asia and Melanesia, with 14 physicians to every 100,000

Table 3–8
Medical and Selected Allied Health Personnel, Various Developing Countries, 1975

Country	Physicians	Medical Assistants	Nurses	Assistant Nurses
Burundi	81	72	140	210
Ethiopia	374	213	892	983
Gambia	19	96	0	0
Ghana	939	260	3,321	3,561
Kenya	766	674	1,578	2,133
Malawi	104	508	365	790
Niger	83	210	558	68
Sudan	1,400	1,794	287	11,670
Bangladesh	5,103	1,034	1,214	1,200
Iraq	4,500	2,383	3,535	3,610
Laos	46	110	42	986
Malasia	107	217	413	324
Nepal	338	692	335	372

Source: World Health Organization, *World Health Statistics Annual, Hospital Personnel and Hospital Establishments*, (Geneva, Switzerland: World Health Organization, 1977) vol. 3 pp. 2–53.

inhabitants, have proportionately to population 11 times fewer physicians than Western Europe.[49]

The density of each category of health worker varies widely from one region of the world to another. Moreover in certain cases it seems that substitution takes place between two professions, the short supply of some being offset by the relatively abundant supply of others. Finally, all the professions considered are not represented in all regions. This indicates the variety that exists in the organization of health-service delivery around the world. In fact the health professions are not mutually independent and relationships of a frequently complex and variable kind develop between their respective frequencies in the population.

Table 3–9 indicates the variations in health manpower between various regions of the world. As the table indicates, health manpower resources vary greatly from one region of the world to another. In addition, there are often considerable disparities between the different parts of a particular country. Within each nation the most striking feature is the divergency in supply between rural and urban areas. For example, in 1970 in Venezuela the rural density amounted to only 31 percent of the urban density. The corresponding figures are 20 percent in Morocco, 11 percent in Nigeria and India, and less than 4 percent in Ethiopia and Nicaragua.[50] In general the poorer the country, the greater disparity in supply of medical manpower between rural and urban areas. Often the increase in total supply of a category of health personnel is manifested only in the towns, while the situation worsens or remains the same in the rural areas.

Table 3–9
Selected Health Workers per 100,000 Inhabitants, 1975

Regions	Medical Workers[a]	Dental Workers[b]	Diagnostic and Research Technicians[c]	Pharmacists	Sanitarians
Middle Africa	52	—	3	1	—
Middle South Africa	59	3	4	9	5
Caribbean	211	19	25	14	9
Temperate South America	294	21	17	10	3
East Asia	394	48	25	63	10
Northern America	817	75	115	63	8
Western Europe	563	44	44	48	3
Eastern Europe	679	62	62	34	14

Source: Bui Dang Ha Doan, "Statistical Analysis of the World Manpower Situation, Circa, 1975," *World Health Statistics Quarterly* 33, no. 2 (1980): 134.
a. Physicians, midwives, nurses, multipurpose health workers.
b. Dentists, dental technicians, and dental operation auxiliaries.
c. Laboratory and radiological technicians and auxiliaries.

As indicated previously, the cost of training auxiliaries is far less than for physicians and dentists. This is illustrated in table 3–10, which indicates the number of health workers that could be trained for the same cost as training one physician in several developing countries.

As is evident, extensive use of health auxiliaries permits considerable savings in training costs. Moreover there is no world market for auxiliaries, so that one does not have to consider the problem of international migration of paramedical personnel.

Foreign Medical Graduates

About 1972 there were at least 140,000 physicians located in countries other than those to which they were nationals or in which they had been born or trained. This figure represented 6 percent of the world's physicians at that time (excluding the People's Republic of China). On average a number equal to one-eighth of the world's production of physicians emigrated annually during the 1970s.[51]

Before World War II, the movement of physicians had generally been from one developed country to another, as well as from the more developed countries to the less developed. During recent years, however, increasing numbers of physicians have been going not only from the less developed to the more developed countries, but also from the poorest to the higher-income developing countries. The shift in the origin of physicians emigrating to the United States is indicated in table 3–11.

Table 3–10
Number of Personnel Produced for Cost of Educating
One Physician, Selected Countries

Country or Region and Health Personnel	Number of Workers Trained for Cost of Educating One Physician
Thailand	
Nurse	5
Auxiliary Sanitarian	19
East Africa	
Nurse	3
Auxiliary sanitarian	15
Medical assistant	20
Auxiliary nurse	30
Colombia	
Nurse	8
Auxiliary nurse	25
Pakistan	
Nurse	4
Medical assistant	24
Lady health visitor	24
Midwife	60
Sanitary inspector	60

Source: Alfonso Mejia, Helena Pizurki, and Erica Royston, *Physician and Nurse Migration: Analysis and Policy Implications* (Geneva, Switzerland: World Health Organization, 1979), p. 149.

The foregoing figures tend to indicate that the migrants from the developing countries are replacing rather than merely supplementing those from developed countries.[52] There is little evidence that the growth in physician migration from Asia represented only an addition to a constant-size stream of migrants from Europe.

In most cases the major increase in migration did not begin until the late 1950s and early 1960s. The first postwar wave of migration was one that physicians shared with other types of laborpower and was in the nature of a large-scale exodus from postwar Europe to the United States and Canada, notably from the Federal Republic of Germany. By 1959 there were 15,000 foreign medical graduates (FMGs) in the United States (excluding Canadians), accounting for 7 percent of physician stock. In 1963 the number had risen to 31,000, accounting for 11 percent of the supply of physicians. The change in immigration laws in 1965 (which abolished the discriminatory national quota system) marked the beginning of the shift in the countries of origin of the FMGs entering the United States but did not really accelerate the growth in the size of the FMG pool. The increase in the number of FMGs employed in the United States occurred later. (See table 3–12.)

In proportional terms, the rate of growth has been declining but in a highly irregular manner. Whereas the number of FMGs in the United States

Table 3-11

Average Number of Physicians Entering the United States, by World Region, 1965-1973

Origin	1965-1969	1970-1973	Change (%)
Europe	1,828	1,561	-15
North and Central America	1,164	1,091	-6
Asia	3,336	3,766	+13
South America	572	776	+33
Africa	233[a]	353	+52
Average, All Countries	7,220[a]	7,664	+6

Source: Alfonso Mejia, Helena Pizurki, and Erica Royston, *Physician and Nurse Migration: Analysis and Policy Implications* (Geneva, Switzerland: World Health Organization, 1979), p. 27.

a. 1967 to 1969 only.

more than doubled from 1963 to 1978, the rate of increase steadily declined. Thus the number of FMGs rose 48 percent from 1963 to 1967, 34 percent from 1970 to 1974, and only 18 percent from 1974-1978.[53]

A declining rate of increase is also reflected in the proportion of FMGs of all physicians. In 1963 FMGs accounted for 11 percent of the total number of physicians. Four years later, the percentage was 15 percent. However, during the 1970s, the proportion of FMGs grew by only 0.7 percent each year from 1971 to 1974, and only 0.2 percent each year from 1974 to 1978. In 1978 there were nearly 84,000 active FMGs who represented 21 percent of the total supply of active physicians.[54]

About one-fifth of migrant physicians entering the United States either return to their homelands or go on to other countries. If one assumes that those who were not located in the United States had returned to the country where they obtained their medical education, this would mean that 27 percent of the Asian graduates, 15 percent of the Latin American graduates, and 13 percent of the European graduates had returned, the overall rate of return being 18 percent.[55]

In general the poorer the country, the greater the magnitude of emigration relative to total domestic supply. Among the 38 countries having a per-capita gross domestic product (GDP) of less than $800 in 1970, some 20 had emigration rates exceeding 10 percent, with some as high as 60 percent or more. However, 6 were net recipients, with some countries experiencing physician gains of over 60 percent. These latter countries were primarily former colonies that did not have sufficient native physicians to replace the number of expatriates who left soon after independence.

Countries in the middle-income range those with a GDP per capita between U.S.$800 and $2,000, experienced some emigration, though usually less than 10 percent of total supply. Once a country attains a GDP per capita of U.S.$2,000 or more, it tends to attract physicians. Only a few countries at this income level experienced net emigration.[56]

Table 3–12
Number of Foreign Medical
Graduates Obtaining Permanent
Immigrant Visas, 1952–1978

Year	Permanent Immigrants
1952	1,201
1955	1,046
1960	1,574
1965	2,012
1970	3,128
1973	3,158
1974	7,119
1974	4,532
1975	5,361
1976	6,184
1977	7,073
1978	4,435

Source: U.S. Department of Health and Human Services, *Third Report to the President and Congress on the Status of Health Professions Personnel in the United States*, DHHS Publication no. (HRA)82-2 (Washington, D.C.: U.S. Department of Health and Human Services, 1982), p. iv–92.

Other things being equal there is a certain sustainable level of physician supply appropriate for each per-capita income level, and those countries in which the total supply is greater than the economy can sustain are likely to experience an outflow of physicians.

While one can maintain that countries with more than the sustainable level should not increase the number of new graduates, it does not automatically follow that cutting medical-school enrollment will cause the emigration rate to fall. For example, in the Philippines a decline in the number of graduates was followed by a fall in the physician/population ratio, rather than by a slowing down of emigration.

In many of the developing countries with larger numbers of new graduates than the economy can absorb, the output of physicians is determined by the demand for medical education, which is itself part of the general demand for higher education. Because of inadequate manpower planning, the enrollment in many fields is completely unrelated to employment opportunities. In countries like India and the Philippines, the number of university graduates has increased far more rapidly than the demand for their services and hence has led to high unemployment among graduates. The relatively high priority placed on higher education in contrast to health is well illustrated by the case of the Philippines, where government health expenditure accounted for 3.2 percent of the national budget in 1974 compared to 13.5 percent for education.

Not only is the economic base of many developing countries insufficient to provide sufficient employment for the physicians being trained there, but the training itself is often irrelevant to the needs of the country in terms of health services. In most countries the medical education provided is geared to meeting the world economic demand for personal health care as opposed to the more pervasive needs of the majority of the population at home. Moreover since the U.S. medical system is specialty oriented, countries that train a disproportionate number of specialists are more likely to lose physicians to developed countries than otherwise. This reflects the fact that the medical-school faculty in many developing countries received their training in highly industrialized nations. Thus their role models were physicians who faced a far different set of medical problems and had far more resources to deal with them than is the case in poor countries.

The simplest method of quantifying losses and gains in monetary terms resulting from the emigration of physicians is to determine the cost of producing or replacing those who migrated. For example, one estimate of the cost of medical education in a developing country is $20,000 compared with $83,000 to train a physician in the United States.[57] If those same values are applied to the number of foreign-trained physicians in the U.S. in 1978 (over 71,000), then this country could be considered as having "saved" nearly $6 billion by importing physicians trained abroad; and the donor countries, as a whole, could be considered as having lost nearly $1.5 billion worth of medical education, assuming that the physicians remain in the United States. However, these figures are underestimates of the cost of medical migration. They do not consider the opportunity cost incurred by the country of origin while the individual was receiving his formal education. This cost is considerable.

Even if the cost of training a physician in a developing country were only $10,000, Haiti's lost investment, in terms of physician manpower, would be $5.2 million compared to a government health budget in 1970 of $3.9 million. In the case of the Philippines, there was a lost investment of $94.5 million against a government health budget of $42.6 million. In the case of South Korea and Iran, the lost investment amounted to more than half the country's government health budget.

A study undertaken by the United Nations' Conference on Trade and Development approached the problem of assessing gains and losses by focusing on the total net income and the imputed capital value of the migrants rather than on the cost of their education. The study is based on the assumption that migrants take with them their productivity and their earning capacity. The recipient countries with which the study deals are Canada, the United Kingdom, and the United States. The study focused on physicians, surgeons, and dentists, a total of 46,408 individuals, who emigrated to these countries from developing nations from 1968 to 1972. According to the findings of the study, the physicians, surgeons, and dentists involved represent a gross imputed capital value of $20.5 billion and a net income gain of $18.75 billion for the three recipient countries combined.[58]

Two closely related suggestions have been made to reduce the flow of physicians to developed countries. The first is to indigenize medical institutions in developing countries. An essential part of this process would be to establish local qualifications that are highly suitable to the medical needs of the local populace and relatively unacceptable to overseas employers. Thus, for instance, medical schools might graduate physicians who know a great deal about preventing the spread of tropical diseases and very little about curing the chronic diseases that are more common in the northern hemisphere.

Second, specialists are more likely to migrate than other practitioners because of the similarity of their training to U.S. medical practice. In addition, these specialists tend to concentrate in urban areas of the developing countries, where the effective demand for their services is low, stimulating emigration due to low practitioner incomes. If foreign medical schools were to concentrate on preparing their graduates for general medical practice, fewer physicians would leave.

Summary

The issue of health manpower shortages has been of major importance in the postwar period. Recent work on measuring shortages has focused on the development of complex mathematical models to determine requirements and supply in selected health occupations. The Graduate Medical Education National Advisory Committee's projections, which are based on this latter approach, forecast a considerable surplus of physicians by 1990 and an even larger surplus by the year 2000.

From 1963 until 1976, health labor legislation encouraged the growth in enrollment of students in health professions training institutions. This reflected the perceived shortage of health labor power. From 1976 to 1983 legislation on health manpower became progressively more restrictive, with many subsidy programs being eliminated.

While the spatial maldistribution of health professionals in the United States remains a problem, there is some evidence that it is becoming less severe. From 1974 to 1978 the most rapid rate of growth in the number of physicians has occurred in those areas with the fewest doctors.

The number of allied health workers in the United States now totals over 3.5 million. The two occupations that have grown most rapidly during the 1970s are physician's assistant and nurse practitioner. There is evidence that utilizing such personnel can increase physicians' productivity and income. However, the expected surplus of physicians in the 1980s and 1990s clouds the future need for these new health practitioners.

In developing countries the need for health auxiliaries is acute because the shortage of health professionals, particularly in the rural areas, is so severe. These are much less expensive to train than physicians, and unlike physicians, are unlikely to emigrate. However, auxiliaries sometimes provide services to patients whom they are not qualified to treat instead of referring the patients elsewhere.

The United States has received a large inflow of foreign medical graduates. These persons, who have increasingly come from developing countries, will account for much of the coming surplus of physicians in the United States. If medical education in developing countries focused on general practice and primary health care, physicians would perhaps be less likely to emigrate. This is particularly the case if the new supply of physicians is not greater than the economy can absorb.

Notes

1. W. Lee Hansen, "An Appraisal of Physician Manpower Projections," *Inquiry* 7, no. 1 (March 1970): 103.

2. C.G. Archibald, "The Factor Gap and the Level of Wages," *Economic Record* 30, no. 59 (November 1954): 188–199.

3. Archibald, "The Factor Gap," p. 189.

4. Roger Lee and Lewis Jones, *The Fundamentals of Good Medical Care* (Chicago: Unversity of Chicago Press, 1933), p. 115.

5. Hyman Schonfeld, Jean Heston, and Isadore Falk, "Number of Physicians Required for Primary Medical Care," *New England Journal of Medicine* 286, no. 11 (May 16, 1972): 574–575.

6. See, for example, the variety of estimates presented in Herbert Klarman, "Economic Aspects of Projecting Requirements for Health Manpower," *Journal of Human Resources* 3, no. 3 (Summer 1969): 365.

7. Rashi Fein, *The Doctor Shortage: An Economic Diagnosis* (Washington, D.C.: The Brookings Institution, 1967), p. 4.

8. Ibid., p. 60.

9. U.S. Department of Health, Education, and Welfare, *Medical Care Costs and Prices* (Washington, D.C.: U.S. Government Printing Office, 1972), p. 43.

10. U.S. Bureau of the Census, 1970 Census of Population, *Occupational Characteristics* (Washington, D.C.: U.S. Government Printing Office, 1973), table 4, p. 145.

11. U.S. Department of Commerce, *Statistical Abstract, 1981* (Washington, D.C.: U.S. Government Printing Office, 1981), pp. 108, 405, and 407.

12. Paul Feldstein and Sander Kelman, "An Econometric Model of the Medical Care Sector," in Herbert Klarman (Ed.), *Empirical Studies in Health Economics* (Baltimore Md.: The Johns Hopkins Press, 1970), p. 186.

13. U.S. Department of Health and Human Services, *Summary Report of the Graduate Medical Education National Advisory Committee*, DHHS Publication no. (HRA)81-651 (Washington, D.C.: U.S. Government Printing Office, 1980).

14. Graduate Medical Education National Advisory Committee, *GMENAC Summary Report to the Secretary, Department of Health and Human Services*, vol. 1 (Washington, D.C.: U.S. Department of Health and Human Services, September 1980), p. 3.

15. Previously enacted legislation had authorized institutional grants to schools of public health for training purposes but provided no federal support for medical education and health manpower development per se.

16. T.G. Grupenhoff and Steven Strickland (Eds.), *Federal Laws: Health, Environment, and Manpower*, Sourcebook Series, vol 1 (Washington, D.C.: The Science and Health Communications Group, 1972), p. 4.

17. Ibid., p. 9.

18. Louise Russell, Blair Bourque, and Carol Burke, *Federal Spending, 1969–1974* (Washington, D.C.: National Planning Association, 1974), p. 28.

19. U.S. Congress, *Congressional Quarterly Almanac, 1976* (Washington, D.C.: U.S. Government Printing Office, 1976), pp. 2685–2687.

20. U.S. Department of Health and Human Services, Public Health Service, *Chronology: Health Professions Legislation, 1956–1979*, DHHS Publication no. (HRA)80-69, p. HB-78 (Washington, D.C.: U.S. Department of Health and Human Services, August 1980).

21. Association of American Medical Colleges, *The Omnibus Budget Reconciliation Act of 1981*, Memorandum 81-37, August 7, 1981, processed attachment II, p. 1.

22. Ibid., attachment II, p. 10.

23. J.E. Weiss, "Socio-Economic and Technological Factors in Trends of Physicians to Specialize," *HSMHA Health Reports* 86, no. 1 (January 1971): 46–51.

24. Graduate Medical Education National Advisory Committee, "Supply and Distribution of Physicians and Physician Extenders," Staff Papers, no. 2, DHEW Publication no. (HRA)78-111, 1978, p. 37.

25. Alan Sorkin, *Health Manpower: An Economic Perspective* (Lexington, Mass.: Lexington Books, D.C. Heath, 1977), p. 107.

26. U.S. Department of Health and Human Services, *Third Report to the President and Congress on the Status of Health Professions Personnel in the United States*, DHHS Publication no. (HRA)82-2 (Washington, D.C.: U.S. Department of Health and Human Services, January 1982), p. IV-25.

27. W.B. Schwartz et al., "The Changing Distribution of Board-Certified Physicians," *New England Journal of Medicine* 303, no. 18 (October 30, 1980): 1032-1038.

28. U.S. Department of Health, Education, and Welfare, "Personnel Training Act of 1966 as Amended," *Report to the President and Congress on the Allied Health Professions* (Washington, D.C.: U.S. Government Printing Office, 1969), p. 1.

29. Sorkin, *Health Manpower*, p. 43; Engin Holmstrom, *The Information Gap in Allied Health Manpower* (Atlanta, Ga.: Southern Regional Education Board, 1981), p. 11.

30. Holmstrom, *Information Gap in Allied Health Manpower,* p. 20.

31. Ibid.

32. Henry Perry and Bina Breitner, *Physician Assistants: Their Contribution to Health Care* (New York: Human Sciences Press, 1982), p. 106; U.S. Department of Health and Human Services, *Third Report to the President and Congress,* p. V-1.

33. Council on Health Manpower, *The Physician's Assistant—A Progress Report* (Chicago: American Medical Association, 1971), p. 16.

34. R.M. Scheffler, "Supply and Demand for New Health Professionals: Physician Assistants and Medex," Bureau of Health Manpower, Department of Health, Education, and Welfare, Contract no. 1-MB-44184, October 1, 1977, p. 7.

35. E.C. Nelson, A.R. Jacobs, P.E. Breer, and K.G. Johnson, "Impact of Physician Assistants on Patient Visits in Ambulatory Care Practices," *Annals of Internal Medicine* 82, no. 5 (May 1975): 608–612.

36. Comptroller General of the United States, *Report to the Congress: Progress and Problems in Training and Use of Assistants to Primary Care Physicians* (Washington, D.C.: U.S. Department of Health, Education, and Welfare, April 8, 1975), p. 33.

37. System Sciences, Inc., *Survey and Evaluation of the Physician Extender Reimbursement Program*, U.S. Department of Health, Education, and Welfare, Contract no. SSA-600-76-0167, Bethesda, Md., March 1978, p. 54.

38. E.C. Nelson, A.R. Jacobs, K. Cordner, and K.G. Johnson, "Financial Impact of Physician Assistants on Medical Practice," *New England Journal of Medicine* 293, no. 11 (September 11, 1975): 529.

39. Perry and Breitner, *Physician Assistants*, pp. 77–78.

40. Perry and Breitner, *Physician Assistants*, p. 81.

41. System Sciences, *Physician Extender Reimbursement Program.*

42. Perry and Breitner, *Physician Assistants,* pp. 123–124.

43. Cited by Doris Storms, *Training and Use of Auxiliary Health Workers: Lessons from Developing Countries*, Monograph no. 3 (Washington, D.C.: American Public Health Association, 1979), p. 9.

44. World Health Organization, "What's in a Name?" *World Health Magazine*, March 1972, p. 27.

45. Maurice King (Ed.), *Medical Care in Developing Countries* (Nairobi: Oxford University Press, 1966), p. 7-2.

46. Storms, *Training and Use of Auxiliary Health Workers*, p. 9.

47. Cited in Ibid., p. 18.

48. King (Ed.), *Medical Care in Developing Countries*, pp. 7-6–7-7.

49. Bui Dang Ha Doan, "Statistical Analysis of the World Health Manpower Situation Area, 1975," *World Health Statistics Quarterly* 33, no. 2 (1980): 130.

50. Ibid., p. 137.

51. A. Mejia, H. Pizurki, and E. Royston, *Physician and Nurse Migration: Analysis and Policy Implications* (Geneva: World Health Organization 1979), p. 24.

52. Ibid., pp. 27–28.

53. U.S. Department of Health and Human Services, *Third Report to the President and Congress*, p. IV-9.

54. Ibid.

55. Mejia et al., *Physician and Nurse Migration*, p. 92.

56. Ibid., p. 105.

57. U.S. Library of Congress, Congressional Research Service, *Brain Drain: A Study of the Persistent Issue of International Mobility* (Washington, D.C.: U.S. Government Printing Office, 1974), p. 152.

58. United Nations' Conference on Trade and Development, *The Reverse Transfer of Technology: Its Dimensions, Economic Effects, and Policy Implications* (Geneva: United Nations Conference on Trade and Development, 1975), p. 39.

4

Hospital Costs and Reimbursement

This chapter focuses on two major issues, the rising cost of hospital care and the methods by which hospitals are reimbursed for services rendered. The interrelationships that exist between hospital costs and reimbursement will also be considered.

Hospital Statistics

The most significant trend data, 1950 to 1980, for nonfederal short-term hospitals are presented in table 4–1. The number of beds per thousand population increased 30 percent over the 30-year period but was virtually unchanged from 1975 to 1980. In-patient admissions rose 117 percent from 1950 to 1980 but rose less than 10 percent from 1975 to 1980. The average length of stay has fluctuated slightly in the period under consideration and was 7.3 percent lower in 1980 as compared to 1950. However, the in-patient population in absolute numbers (average daily census) has continued to rise and reached 748,000 in 1980.

Out-patient care is an increasingly important hospital activity. Unfortunately, complete data are not available for these services. However, incomplete statistics indicate a steep rise, especially in emergency room and private diagnostic services. From 1957 to 1980 out-patient visits increased from 67 million to 207 million—a gain of 209 percent. This was nearly 50 percent more rapid than the rate of increase in hospital admissions, and it indicates some degree of substitution of outpatient care for inpatient care.[1]

Full-time personnel (or their equivalents in part-time workers) rose 335 percent from 1950 to 1980 and totaled 2.88 million in 1980. The personnel-patient ratio rose 88 percent to a 1980 high of 3.3 employees per patient. In spite of the increase in personnel and higher wages and salaries, payroll as a percentage of total expenses declined steadily after 1970, and in 1980 was less than one-half of total costs.

Total expense per patient day, the hospital's average per-diem cost, rose very rapidly from 1950 to 1980—a total of 1,705 percent to a level of $281.92. The slight decline in length of stay was more than offset by cost increases, and the average expense per patient stay rose 1,783 percent to $2,141.59.

Table 4-1
U.S. Nonfederal Short-Term Hospitals—Selected Data, 1950–1980

	1950	1960	1970	1975	1980	Percentage Increase		
						1950–1980	1960–1970	1970–1980
Total civilian resident population (millions)	150.8	178.2	205.1	216.0	227.7	51.0	15.1	11.0
Number of hospitals	5,031	5,407	5,859	5,979	5,904	17.4	8.3	0.7
Number of beds (thousands)	505	639	848	947	992	96.4	32.7	17.0
Beds per 1,000 population	3.35	3.59	4.14	4.38	4.36	30.1	15.3	1.1
Admissions (thousands)	16,663	22,970	29,252	33,519	36,198	117.2	27.3	23.7
Admissions per 1,000 population	110.5	128.9	142.6	155.2	159.0	43.9	10.6	11.5
Average daily census (thousands)	372	477	622	708	748	101.1	38.8	20.3
Patient days per 1,000 population	895	980	1,169	1,195	1,199	34.0	19.3	-2.6
Occupancy (%)	73.7	74.7	78.0	74.8	75.4	2.3	4.4	-3.3
Average length of stay (days)	8.1	7.6	8.2	7.7	7.6	-6.2	7.9	-7.3
Total expenses ($ millions)	2,120	5,617	19,560	39,110	76,970	3,530.1	248.2	293.5
Total expenses per patient day	15.62	32.23	81.58	151.51	281.92	1,704.9	153.1	245.6
Expenses per patient stay	127.26	244.53	668.96	1,166.62	2,142.59	1,783.6	173.6	220.3
Expenses per patient stay (1980 $)	435.81	680.52	1,419.06	1,786.23	2,142.59	391.6	108.6	51.0
Expense per person	14.06	31.52	95.37	181.06	338.03	2,304.1	202.6	254.4
Expense per person (1980 $)	48.26	87.72	202.31	277.22	338.03	600.4	130.6	67.1
Full-time personnel (thousands)[a]	662	1,080	1,929	2,399	2,879	334.9	78.6	49.2
Full-time personnel per 100 patients[a]	178	226	265	298	334	87.6	17.2	26.0
Payroll expenses ($ millions)	1,203	3,400	11,421	20,749	37,460	3,013.8	226.4	228.0
Payroll expenses per patient day	8.86	20.08	47.63	79.00	137.76	1,454.8	137.2	189.2
Payroll expenses per patient day (1980 $)	30.35	55.86	101.04	120.96	137.76	353.9	80.9	36.3
Average payroll expense per employee	1,817	3,229	5,921	8,649	13,011	616.1	82.8	119.7
Payroll expense as percentage of total expense	56.7	62.3	58.4	53.1	48.7	-14.1	-6.3	-16.6

Source: American Hospital Association, *Hospital Statistics, 1981* (Chicago: American Hospital Association, 1980), p. 5.
a. Includes part-time-equivalents except in 1950.

An important indicator of changing hospital operations, not shown in table 4–1, is the rising number of institutions with specialized technical facilities. Virtually all nonfederal short-term hospitals have a clinical laboratory and diagnostic x-ray equipment compared with 76 and 86 percent, respectively, in 1946. The percentage of hospitals with registered pharmacists increased from 63 percent in 1967 to 96 percent in 1980.[2]

Types of Hospitals

There are a number of different kinds of hospitals. As indicated earlier, this chapter does not consider long-term hospitals. Moreover federal hospitals will be excluded from analysis because they are not generally accessible to the public. Even within the designation "nonfederal short-term," there are numerous classifications. The 1980 distribution according to ownership and relative size is as follows:[3]

	Percentage		
	Hospitals	*Beds*	*Full-Time Personnel*
Voluntary	56.6	69.9	72.5
Proprietary	12.4	8.8	6.6
State and local government	31.0	21.3	20.9
Total, nonfederal short-term	100.0	100.0	100.0

The state and local hospitals are owned and operated by municipalities, counties, or states. In heavily populated or urbanized areas they tend to serve mainly the indigent and low-income patients. Charges have been traditionally related to income. However, in some localities, the county hospital is the only hospital within a broad geographic area and serves the entire population.

The proprietary hospital is a business enterprise, usually owned and operated by groups of doctors in connection with their medical practice but sometimes as a separate business activity. Such hospitals may also be owned by other private investors.[4] Increasingly corporations are operating nationwide chains of proprietary hospitals, raising the possibility of increasing seller concentration in this phase of the hospital industry.

The proprietary hospitals are guided primarily by profit considerations in determining the range of services offered and the prices to be charged for these services. Thus they exhibit behavior similar to private firms in other industries and attempt to maximize profits. Generally these hospitals limit their services to full-pay patients and avoid the medically indigent. However, with the government paying full "reasonable costs" under Medicare, on behalf of the aged poor, proprietary hospitals have increased the proportion of low-income elderly patients.

The voluntary hospital is neither a public enterprise nor is it a profit-making institution. Ownership is vague, as the original capital is usually raised through community drives or philanthropy.[5] A substantial number are controlled by Catholic and other religious groups. The voluntary hospital is legally operated by a board of trustees, usually composed of prominent community figures.

Some of the nonprofit aspects of the voluntary hospital are disappearing. The charity patient is more likely to go elsewhere, and because of Medicaid and Medicare, there are fewer charity patients. Increasingly the voluntary hospital expects to be paid at least at the level of costs for services rendered. Both proprietary and voluntary hospitals hope to produce a profit, in the sense that current operating revenues will exceed costs. The difference between them lies in what is done with the surplus. None of the voluntary hospitals' surplus can be distributed to the "owners"; it is all ultimately reinvested in expansion, renovation, or improvement.

Because the voluntary hospital is predominant in the American hospital system, most of the subsequent analysis of hospital costs and reimbursement focuses on these institutions.

The doctor's relationship to the hospital has become increasingly complex as the hospital's role in professional life has become more important. Although the degree of his association varies with the type of practice, probably at least 50 percent of the average physician's income is earned in the hospital. A surgeon or radiologist may earn up to 100 percent of his income there. In any case, while the physician is the key and indispensable figure in the hospital, with wide authority and latitude, he is not part of the administrative or financial structure. Moreover a united and determined medical staff can effectively take over a hospital and operate it without any of the financial risks or responsibilities that it otherwise would face.

Hospital Expenditures

In the recent past hospital expenditures have grown rapidly. From 1968 to 1979 community hospital expenditures per adjusted admission increased at an average annual rate of 12 percent, and total community hospital expenditures increased at an average annual rate of 15 percent. This growth has been more rapid than that of consumer prices for the economy as a whole.

Consumer prices increased at an average annual rate of approximately 6 percent during the 1968–1979 period, while total personal consumption expenditures rose at an annual rate of 10 percent.

Federal outlays for hospital care under the Medicare and Medicaid programs, which together presently account for about 40 percent of community hospital revenues, have increased even more rapidly. From 1968 to 1978 their annual rate of increase averaged 17 percent.

In the absence of effective hospital cost containment, hospital expenditures are projected by the Congressional Budget Office to nearly double between fiscal year 1979 and fiscal year 1984.[6] Annual expenditures will increase by about $63 billion (from $66 to $129 billion) over the period, while federal Medicare and Medicaid outlays for hospital care are expected to increase by about $31 billion (from $23 billion to $54 billion).

As expenditures rise, taxes or deficits must increase to meet the correspondingly higher outlays from federal health programs, while business and individuals must pay higher premiums for health-insurance plans. Fewer resources are available for other types of private and public consumption.

However, reallocation of resources from one sector to another is typical in a dynamic economy. More resources are allocated to the computer industry each year, for example. Why then is there a concern about additional resources flowing into the hospital sector?

The concern stems from doubts about whether the increases in expenditures have resulted in concomitant gains in the value of medical services. Many experts claim that too many resources are being allocated to health services in general and hospital care in particular. They assert that there is waste partially caused by duplication of facilities and poor management and that some services have little or no effectiveness and thus are unnecessary. Technical ignorance on the part of patients, and the fact that much medical expense is borne by third parties such as governments and insurance companies, cause competition to be weaker in the health sector than in other markets. Since the patient frequently does not pay directly for services rendered, the normal market test—whether a service can be sold at a given price—is not applicable.

Components of Hospital Expenditure Increases

Hospital expenditure increases are made up of four basic components:[7]

1. The higher prices hospitals pay for the goods and services used in the delivery of care. These hospital inputs include food, fuel supplies, labor, and capital goods.

2. The increased use of hospital services. The number of hospital admissions and days of hospital care have been rising. Outpatient visits have also been increasing very rapidly.
3. The changing character—often referred to as the "service intensity"—of hospital services. Hospitals continually add services and deliver existing ones (for example, lab tests and x-rays) more frequently.
4. Slow productivity increases. Private firms rely on productivity gains to keep increases in product prices below gains in wages. If hospital productivity advances relative to wage increases are smaller than in other industries, prices of hospital services and expenditures on hospital care will increase more rapidly than expenditures in other sectors.

Although increases in the prices of hospital inputs account for over half of the growth in hospital expenditures, increases in utilization and intensity have been responsible for the remaining rapid increase in total outlays for hospital services. Surprisingly, wage increases among hospital workers have not been an important cause of hospital inflation in recent years.

For example, a recent study compared gains in hospital employee real wages to wage gains of workers of similar quality in other sectors. It was found that during the 1960s hospital workers' real wages rose faster than those of comparable employee groups. However, during the 1970s hospital workers' wages failed to keep pace with other workers of similar quality; in fact wages of hospital workers even failed to keep pace with inflation.[8]

Factors other than wage and price increases account for almost all of the portion of hospital expenditure increases that exceeded the growth in spending in the economy as a whole. Hospital utilization increased faster than the amount that could be explained by the growth and aging of the population. As measured by adjusted admissions (a measure combining admissions and out-patient visits), utilization increased at an average annual rate of 2.8 percent. Meanwhile population (adjusted for the higher utilization associated with the aging of the population) grew by only 1.3 percent a year. Net intensity increased at an average annual rate of 3.2 percent. (See table 4–2.)

Hospital labor intensity per patient day increased by 19 percent between 1971 and 1978. On the average, hospitals employed 272 persons per 100 patients in 1970 and 323 employees per 100 patients in 1978. Real assests per bed grew by 28 percent and real assets per 1,000 population increased by 37 percent during the period 1971–1977. Moreover the American Hospital Association's intensity index rose by 55.4 percent during the period January 1970 to October 1979. This index measures the quantities of 37 hospital inputs provided per typical patient day, such as lab tests, x-rays, prescriptions, operating room visits, and nursing manhours weighted by base year costs.[9]

Table 4–2
Components of Annual Increases in Hospital Expenditures, 1968–1979 (%)

Calendar Year	Price of Hospital Inputs	Utilization	Itensity	Total
1969	5.9	2.2	8.3	17.2
1970	6.7	6.4	3.5	17.5
1971	4.9	0.6	5.2	11.0
1972	5.0	3.2	3.5	12.1
1973	6.3	4.2	1.1	12.0
1974	14.4	3.9	−2.5	16.0
1975	11.0	1.1	4.7	17.5
1976	7.4	3.9	6.7	19.1
1977	7.6	2.9	4.4	15.6
1978	8.0	0.8	3.6	12.8
1979	10.1	1.7	1.3	13.4
Average annual increase	7.9	2.8	3.2	14.9

Source: Congressional Budget Office, *Controlling Rising Hospital Costs* (Washington, D.C.: U.S. Government Printing Office, 1979), p. 5; and U.S. Department of Health, Education, and Welfare, *Health: United States, 1980* (Washington, D.C.: U.S. Government Printing Office, 1980), p. 102.

Causes of Rapid Expenditure Increases

Four major reasons have been suggested to explain why hospital expenditures have been growing more rapidly than can be accounted for by the increased prices of hospital inputs and by population increases: a lack of competition in the market for hospital services, new technological developments, rising real incomes, and the changing health status of the population.[10] Changing consumer tastes and preferences, while difficult to precisely specify, also affect the growth in hospital expenditures.

Lack of Competition

The hospital industry is much less competitive than other industries. Since over 90 percent of hospital bills are paid for by third parties such as Medicare, Medicaid, and private insurance companies, patients usually have little immediate financial interest in the cost of their care. Further, few patients or doctors have much information as to whether particular services delivered by a hospital are worth their cost; a situation probably made worse by the extensiveness of third-party payment.

Health insurance raises the demand for hospital care in two ways. From the perspective of the patient, the net price of hospital care is reduced so that financial deterrence declines. Thus for a given illness, patients are less reluctant to be hospitalized and to remain there. They are more likely to insist that their physicians employ all the diagnostic or therapeutic procedures available. With the physician acting on behalf of the patient, insurance gives strong inducements to order additional services. It removes a deterrent to the ordering of any service that might benefit the patient regardless of cost. Moreover under the fee-for-service system of financing, insurance increases the additional income physicians may obtain from performing additional services. Since the balancing of costs and benefits of additional services is less likely to occur, insurance results in higher and more rapidly rising expenditures on hospital care than would occur in its absence.

Increased demand for medical care associated with greater insurance coverage can cause increases in service intensity. As the net price to the patient declines, individuals demand higher quality care and more amenities such as better food, more nurses, and superior accommodations. The increasing insurance coverage, by reducing the price elasticity of demand, allows the provider to charge higher prices without reducing total utilization. The new revenues may then be used to obtain new equipment, hire more staff, and improve patient amenities.

Present tax laws worsen the situation by the way in which health insurance is treated. The exclusion from taxable income of all employer contributions to employee health plans gives employees a strong incentive to sacrifice money wages for more extensive insurance coverage than they would purchase with after-tax dollars. The additional insurance further reduces incentives to economize in the use of medical services. Furthermore, where employers offer a choice of health plans, as for example, between traditional insurance and enrollment in a less expensive health-maintenance organization (HMO), employees usually do not benefit financially from choosing the low-cost plan, thus reducing incentives to choose such plans.

Although hospitals traditionally have shown little concern about the prices charged patients, they do worry about attracting physicians who are the source of patient admissions. Since physicians prefer to practice at hospitals that offer a full range of modern services, hospitals often duplicate each others' facilities. This often results in excess capacity and resultant inefficiency.

Technological Developments

The adoption of new technologies has also contributed to rising expenditures on hospital care. One recent innovation, the coronary bypass operation, costs $10,000 or more. Another, electronic fetal monitoring, is now performed in roughly half of obstetrical cases at a total cost of over $400 million per year. While new technology usually benefits patients and increases hospital productivity, it is often embodied in new services that are additions to, rather than replacements for, existing services. Consequently new technology often increases the utilization of hospital care, an important factor in the growth of expenditures by hospitals.

An important issue is the relationship between the introduction of cost-increasing technology and third-party payment. It is maintained that third-party payment has increased the rate of adoption of such technology. If this is correct, then much of the increase in hospital expenditures associated with new technology is another manifestation of the third-party financing system. However, an alternative position is that technological advances are exogenous, or not influenced by insurance. Indeed the possibility exists that expensive third-party financing is a response to technological developments that have made hospital care more costly.

Rising Personal Income

As people's real incomes grow, they tend to purchase more goods and services of all kinds. Some, especially the uninsured, may demand more hospital care as their incomes rise. Others may purchase more health insurance, leading in turn to increased expenditures for hospital care. However, with over 90 percent of hospital bills already covered by insurance, rising incomes have little additional potential to increase hospital expenditures.

Changing Health Status

Trends in the population's health status also influence expenditures through changes in the utilization and intensity of hospital care. The aging of the population should increase both utilization and intensity. Changing lifestyles may also affect health status and hospital expenditures. However, increasing education and better nonhospital medical care may improve health and reduce in-patient hospital use.

**Cost Differences between Hospitals—
Some Technical Issues**

One of the technical issues that have arisen in studies of hospital costs is the problem of how to define hospital output. The total output of a hospital is usually measured by patient days. It can also be measured by admissions, discharges, or the average daily census. Hospitals produce several different

types of services, including in-patient care, out-patient care, and educational services (teaching and research). Within each of these categories,
these are wide variations among hospitals in the specific types of ouput
produced. Thus regarding inpatient care, it is recognized that the diagnostic
mix of cases differs considerably between hospitals. In order to account for
this in statistical cost functions of hospitals (a cost function indicates the
relationship between total cost and output), several different kinds of
case-mix variables have been used. These include percentages of patients in
various diagnostic categories, case-mix indexes derived from these percentages, and variables indicating the presence or absence of specific types of
treatment facilities and services. Whether these approaches deal adequately
with the problem of output heterogenity is questionable, since even within
specific diagnostic categories there is often variation in the severity of
medical problems. Moreover in the case of out-patient and educational
services, efforts to control for output heterogenity have been more unso-
phisticated.[11]

For both hospital and medical services, there is some likelihood that the
quality of services differs among providers. Since the ability to measure
quality differences is quite limited, one cannot rule out quality differences as
a partial explanation for apparent differences in efficiency among providers.

Statistical cost functions have also been used to study the efficiency of
specific hospital departments (laundry, laboratory, radiology).[12] The focus
has been on the economies of scale, since the existence of substantial scale
economies would argue for the sharing, contracting out, or regionalization
of these departmental activities. The problem of output heterogenity is
obviously less serious in this situation than is the case where the entire
hospital is the focus of investigation. There is probably less heterogeneity
across hospitals in an output measure such as pounds of laundry processed
than in a measure such as patient days.

Hospital Reimbursement

Three basic methods have been used to determine the level of reimbursement made by third-party payers to hospitals. These are reimbursement on
the basis of (1) charges, (2) costs, and (3) prospective reimbursement. The
strength and weaknesses of each reimbursement approach will be discussed
in turn.

Charges. A declining share of hospital services is paid for on the basis of
charges determined by the hospital. Patients lacking insurance coverage
(self-pay patients), most commercial insurance carriers, and twenty-seven
of the seventy-four Blue Cross plans across the country (representing 30

percent of total Blue Cross enrollment), reimburse on the basis of charges.[13] This reimbursement mechanism is analogous to the fee-for-service system used by physicians. A hospital first decides which units of service are to be priced separately and then determines its charges based on expected volume relative to operating costs, bad debts and free care, depreciation and interest on existing debt, and finally a margin for expansion and new technology.

Strengths. First, charges are determined prior to the consumption of services and are based on the hospital's expectations about future costs and levels of outputs. At least in the short-run the burden of input price increases or other cost rising factors is absorbed by the hospital rather than the patient or the third party.[14] In addition, consumers can determine prior to discharge what their financial liability will be per billed unit. This is less of an advantage in this particular industry because the number and type of units in the complete illness episode is highly uncertain a priori and strongly affected by the attending physician. Moreover because the hospital is assured of receiving additional revenue for every service that is consumed, it has no incentive to constrain the availability of required services because of financial limitations. From the standpoint of quality of care, this may be an important consideration. Finally, unlike average total cost reimbursement, payment is at least somewhat related to services rendered.

Weaknesses. The first problem comes from the likelihood that not all purchasers of care pay the full cost of services provided to them or to their beneficiaries. Thus the payments made by other purchasers of care must be raised to cover these deficits.

There are believed to be two types of cross-subsidization in hospitals: subsidization across payer groups[15] and subsidization across individual charge-paying patients. Decisions by Medicare or Blue Cross to exclude a portion of teaching costs or to reduce the amount of allowable depreciation expenses, for example, need not cause a lower level of hospital costs to the overall community, but only a change in their distribution.

With respect to subsidization across charge-paying patients, it is widely believed that hospitals systematically set prices above costs for some services and use the resulting surpluses to fund deficits resulting from below-cost pricing for other services.[16] To the extent that the patients who receive the former services do not receive the latter, some subsidization across patients occurs.

Costs. The remaining forty-seven Blue Cross plans (representing 70 percent of total Blue Cross enrollment) and Medicare and Medicaid, all determine reimbursement on the basis of costs incurred in the provision of services to their respective beneficiaries. In recent years these three types of third-party providers have in the aggregate accounted for approximately two-thirds of community-hospital revenue.[17]

In general cost reimbursement is based on the retrospectively determined costs of providing service. It is generally paid as an average per-diem rate. Periodic outlays are made throughout the payment period on the basis of projected costs and volume with an end-of-period adjustment for differences between projected per-diem costs and actual costs.

Excluded costs are those that are unrelated to patient care, such as the costs associated with the gift shop, the cafeteria, and the parking lot. In addition, medical research costs are typically excluded. Bad debts and the costs of free care are not covered by Blue Cross plans, and Medicare reimburses only for the bad debts of its own beneficiaries.[18]

Although depreciation of existing plant and equipment and interest payments on borrowed capital are allowable costs, specific contributions to an internal fund for future capital expenditures (analogous to retained earnings in a for-profit firm) are not made. Instead many Blue Cross plans add an additional factor to costs that generally ranges between 2 and 8 percent. Medicare originally added an extra 2 percent to costs but eliminated it in 1969.

The results of cost-function studies can be useful in setting policies for retrospective (cost-based) reimbursement systems. The fact that hospitals produce many different types of output poses a major problem for third-party payers (such as Medicare) under these systems, because it requires an allocation of each hospital's costs between these different types of output. For example, the determination of a reimbursable cost per patient day requires that nursing costs for out-patient treatment be separated from nursing costs for in-patient treatment.

One method of dealing with this problem is by applying simple apportionment rules. Thus in-patient nursing costs might be computed as total nursing costs multiplied by the ratio of nursing hours assigned to in-patient service as compared to total nursing hours. Similarly in-patient x-ray costs could be calculated as total x-ray costs multiplied by the ratio of in-patient to total films. However, in certain instances, the use of apportionment rules is unhelpful, as in the case where two different types of output are produced simultaneously. The most important example of this is the joint production of education and of patient care in teaching hospitals. While attempts have been made to allocate trainees' time between service and education (as a basis for cost apportionment), it is not possible to draw this distinction in cases where the two activities are carried out simultaneously.[19]

However, statistical cost functions can be used for determining reimbursable costs in the case of joint production. By computing a statistical cost function, for example, from a sample of teaching and nonteaching hospitals, which includes measures of teaching activity (e.g., full-time-equivalent residents) as independent variables, it is possible to estimate the costs that teaching institutions would have incurred in producing their patient-care output if they had provided no educational services. This estimate could in principle be used as the basis for determining reimbursable costs per day.

However, there are a number of important practical problems with this procedure. Estimates of teaching costs have been obtained from several studies, but problems in controlling for other determinants of cost (such as case-mix) have probably introduced bias into these estimates.[20] Further refinements in technique need to be developed, although the existing studies have produced some interesting findings such as that teaching programs may actually permit some types of services to be produced at lower costs.

Strengths of Cost-Based Reimbursement. The use of cost-reimbursement contracts is by no means limited to the hospital industry. Cost contracts are found in development, research, and consulting activities, and in many other areas where the precise characteristics of a product to be purchased are difficult to specify a priori. This type of contracting is utilized because of its flexibility: product specifications can be changed during the contracting period without expensive and time-consuming renegotiations of product price. In addition it provides the maximum incentive for high-quality output. The producer is never induced to make quality trade-offs to lower production costs unless explicitly requested to do so by the purchaser. Finally the burden of increasing cost trends is borne by the purchaser.

Weaknesses. Reasonable cost reimbursement is generally criticized as being highly inflationary and generally inefficient.[21] The rationale for this criticism is that if hospitals are assured of being reimbursed for all incurred costs, there is little or not incentive to reduce costs through increased efficiency, and they are encouraged to use the most sophisticated technology available, even if not medically necessary.

One of the greatest problems in implementing a cost-based reimbursement system is the determination of which costs are allowable and how to measure them. Each system has a set of rules detailing which costs will be reimbursed and how allowable costs are to be defined and computed. These rule differences often raise equity issues. If Medicare disallows a particular component of capital costs because of a restrictive definition of depreciation, will the hospital simply add those costs onto the bills of other patients?

Another problem with this type of reimbursement is the cost of monitoring hospital performance. To assure that payment rules are followed, most third parties undertake at least some cost monitoring. This may be limited only to receiving detailed cost reports or periodic audits, or it may be more extensive. In any case, with large number of service providers, the costs of these monitoring activities can be large and must be included in the cost of this kind of reimbursement.[22]

Prospective Reimbursement

The rapid increase in hospital costs during the 1960s and early 1970s can be attributed in part to the methods by which hospitals were paid. Cost reimbursement and charges reimbursement are inherently inflationary in that they do not provide incentives for cost containment. Recognizing this, government agencies and third-party payers are now experimenting with alternative approaches to reimbursement that incorporate such incentives.

Prospective reimbursement—or more accurately, prospective budget- or rate-setting and reimbursement—is a method of paying hospitals, in which (1) amounts or rates of payment are established in advance for the coming year and (2) hospitals are paid these amounts or rates regardless of the costs they actually incur.[23]

Prospective reimbursement shifts some of the risk for costs from third-party payers to hospitals, in contrast to retrospective cost reimbursement, where payers assume the risk for whatever hospitals spend. Incentives operate in several ways. First, hospitals are motivated to anticipate and justify future expenditures and to establish the need for new facilities and services in attempting to gain recognition of the cost of their plans and its effect on their prospective rates. This could lead to greater cost consciousness in capital and operations planning. Second, hospitals are motivated to identify and monitor the cost implications of the quantity, quality, and scope of services they provide in order to assure themselves that they can operate within their rates. This could lead to improved forecasting, budgeting, cost-finding, and cost-control techniques. Third, hospitals have incentives to keep their actual costs below their rates to avoid losses or to achieve surpluses. This could lead to more effective and efficient operations.

Payment Unit

If a prospective reimbursement scheme uses the hospital budget, departmental budgets, or capitation as the basis of payment, hospitals would have an incentive to limit increases in or reduce both the number of cases treated and the length of stay of hospitalized patients. This is because once the amounts to be paid under these payment units are determined, they would not be affected by admissions or patient days of care provided.

In addition to the incentives to reduce admission and patient days, these payment units provide an incentive for hospitals to contain increases in costs by changing the composition of patients treated and by altering the nature of services provided them. Hospitals might admit fewer individuals with serious conditions, thereby shifting toward a less costly case mix. Hospitals could reduce the scope, quality, and intensity of service that they provide. Each of these actions tends to limit increases in expenditures for equipment, personnel, and supplies and hence should help to keep actual costs below prospective budget or aggregate capitation payment levels.

An incentive also exists for hospitals to improve efficiency, both by increasing input productivity and by shifting toward a less costly input mix. In addition, assuming that hospitals have some buying power, they might resist increases in input prices. The overall effect of using any of the three aforementioned payment units should be a reduction in both the quantity and cost per unit of hospital services, so that total hospital costs should be reduced.[24]

One difference between the hospital budget and departmental budget payment units is that the latter focuses attention on departments where costs or productivity differ from the average. In addition, departmental budgets could be used for deparments over which the administrator has the greatest control, and cost or some other form of reimbursement used for the other departments.

Basing reimbursement on the episode of illness, which would require that a hospital be associated with a medical group or health plan, would bring about the same responses as three payments units discussed before. However, the problem of defining episodes of illness is substantial.

Payment units based on specific services, the case, or the day, are all output related. Thus payment of a fixed amount per case would motivate hospitals to admit more patients; but would encourage them to admit fewer complex cases in order to shorten stays, and to reduce the scope and intensity of services provided.

Admission selectivity could be discouraged by establishing different prospective reimbursement rates for different case types. For example, hospitals treating persons with less expensive conditions would be rewarded only if their costs for those particular conditions were relatively low.

Payment of a fixed amount per day would motivate hospitals to increase the days of care provided, by increasing admissions or lengths of stay, and to shift from more costly to less costly days by admitting patients with less complicated conditions and by reducing the intensity and breadth of services provided.[25]

Reimbursement of fixed amounts for specific services (nursing care, laboratory tests, surgical procedures, x-rays) would encourage hospitals to increase services. Admissions and length of stay might be increased, and hospitals might attempt to admit patients with relatively complex conditions, since they need the most services.

Hospital preferences for the different payment units (in terms of prospective reimbursement) would depend in part on their expectations about future demand. If an increase in utilization is expected, the output-related payment units would be preferred; if a decrease is expected, the budget or capitation payment units would be desired.

Alternative Budget- or Rate-Setting Methods

It has been argued that the impact of prospective reimbursement (positive or negative) depends largely on the payment unit used. Choice of the method used to control or determine the amount to be paid per unit depends upon the ability of alternative methods to establish fair but tight payment levels.

A number of reimbursement methods have been developed. These include the use of multiple-regression equations, the negotiated-budget approach, the percentage-of-mean approach, and the formula approach.

Regression analysis permits estimation of a cost function for all hospitals or for each group of hospitals. The regression coefficients are used in conjunction with the hospital's particular values for the independent variables to yield a reimbursement rate for each institution. This approach has the advantage of allowing continuous adjustment for variables affecting cost, and it is relatively inexpensive to administer. However, the method has the disadvantage that agreement on the appropriate mathematical form of the regression is lacking, especially regarding which independent variables should be included.

The negotiated-budget method considers each hospital separately. Direct negotiations between hospitals and rate-setting organizations thus enable differences among hospitals to be recognized. However, in such meetings, bargaining power is important. For example, in an area with a large number of hospitals, a representative of the rate-setting agency might state, "If I can get a service from other nearby hospitals for this amount, that is the maximum amount you will receive even if your costs are higher." However, in an area with only one hospital, the representative of the rate-setting agency might have less power. In any case the negotiated-budget approach allows a hospital to attempt to gain recognition of its financial requirements and rate setters to minimize the amount allocated for hospital costs, particularly if this seems inordinately high.

The effectiveness of the budget review and approval method of rate setting ultimately depends on the expertise of the rate-setting organization. Careful analysis requires detailed capital and operating budgets and departmental or program review. Projected utilization levels must be examined, and the appropriateness of the quantities and types of resources budgeted to accommodate these use levels must be considered.

The percentage-of-mean approach basically establishes the reimbursement level as some function of the average experience of all similar hospitals. As has been pointed out by Lave, Lave, and Silverman, this approach induces hospitals with below-average costs to raise costs, as well as encouraging high-cost hospitals to reduce costs; the resulting upward trend of the group mean over time reduces system savings.[26]

Formula methods of prospective reimbursement that apply averages, ceilings, price indexes, or projections of the past trends in costs, ignore some of the basic causes of cost differences among hospitals. Thus they may not fully account for changes from year to year in case mix, facilities and services, or utilization levels. Formula methods are more sensitive if cost functions or point systems are employed in which the characteristics of individual hospitals influence their rates. Rates based on a determination of the reasonable costs of producing specific services explicitly disregard the cost differences among individual hospitals.

Some Technical Issues in Prospective Reimbursement

In attempting to set prospective rates for hospitals, regulating commissions or agencies are faced with a number of empirical questions that have in fact been addressed by economists in studies of hospital costs. Three specific issues that have been addressed in cost studies are especially relevant to prospective rate setting: the cost implications of differences in case mix, geographical variations in the factors determining costs, and the relationship of short-run marginal cost to average cost.

The existence of large differences in case mix between hospitals is a potential problem in setting prospective rates because of the related inter-hospital differences in costs. Hospitals that treat many severe or complicated medical problems will generally have a higher average cost (per day or per admission) than hospitals that treat mostly routine cases. If the procedure used for determining rates does not adequately recognize this fact, hospitals treating more severe cases may have an incentive to change their case mix so that they treat fewer of these patients. Another possible strategy is to allow the service quality to deteriorate. Thus if rates are constrained to be at or below some criterion of reasonability (say, the eightieth percentile cost level), which is the same for all hospitals, those that treat mainly complex cases are definitely at a disadvantage. Rate setters have a number of ways to deal with this problem, such as grouping hospitals and setting a different upper limit for each group, or setting upper limits for many specific types of services (laboratory, radiology, recovery room) rather than for an average in-patient day or case. However, what is ultimately required, in order to develop or evaluate any particular rate-setting scheme, is information on the cost implicaiton of case-mix differences.[27]

Hospital cost studies illustrate several different approaches for obtaining this information. One method is to include case-mix descriptors as independent variables in statistical cost functions. The most cumbersome approach is to employ variables describing the percentages of admissions or patient days that fall into different diagnostic categories. A more efficient method is to construct a variable representing a case-mix index that reflects these percentages. In determining the index, greater weight is given to problems requiring specialized treatment, with appropriate facilities being found in only one or two hospitals in an area. A recent empirical test of such an index has shown it to be a very important determinant of costs.[28] In either of the foregoing approaches, the coefficients of the case-mix variables in a statistical cost function can be used to calculate differences in case mix. If this procedure indicates, for example, that the rates established for various hospitals do not adequately reflect these differences in cost, a change in the rate-setting policy (to avoid unfair treatment of hospitals with a costly case mix) may be appropriate.

The reasons for considering geographic differences in the factors influencing cost, in regard to prospective rate setting, are similar to the reasons for being concerned with differences in case mix. Since these factors are beyond the control of the hospital, and if hospitals in high-cost and low-cost areas are subjected to the same rate limitations, then those in low-cost areas are arbitrarily permitted to produce higher-quality services or to operate less efficiently. In order to determine the magnitude of this problem in regard to prospective reimbursement, information obtained from statistical cost functions may again be useful.

In particular, cost functions have been developed with dichotomous variables indicating type of location to determine the cost implications of being located in an urban versus a suburban or rural area. An alternative approach is to include measures of the geographic factors affecting costs (such as wage levels, construction-cost levels, food prices) directly in the cost function. The geographic differences in costs derived from these statistical studies can be compared to the differentials provided for by the rate-setting process to determine whether rate differentials make insufficient or excessive allowance for such spatial factors affecting costs.

The relationship of short-run marginal cost to average cost is important in prospective rate setting because of the need to adjust prospective rates for variations in the volume of output. (See figure 4–1.) If hospitals receive a fixed per-diem rate that is higher than the short-run marginal cost of a patient day, they have an incentive to increase their volume of patient days. However, if the fixed per-diem rate is equal to or less than short-run marginal cost, hospitals will be unable to cover their fixed costs. Thus in order to provide adequate reimbursement for fixed costs while limiting the incentive to increase patient days, a downward rate adjustment for volume

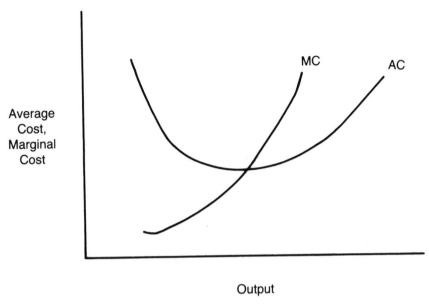

Figure 4–1. Relationship of Short-Run Marginal Cost to Short-Run Average Cost

increases is required. For example, if the basic per-diem rate is set for some target volume, then the rate-setting agency can eliminate the incentive to increase patient days by paying hospitals only 50 percent of the basic rate for patient days in excess of target volume. Obviously the ratio of short-run marginal cost to average cost is a key magnitude in designing this type of rate system,[29] and estimates of this magnitude have been made in a number of hospital cost studies.

Empirical Studies of Prospective Reimbursement

The studies show considerable differences in results. O'Donoghue's estimate for Indiana is a saving of $200 million from 1968 to 1973.[30] The Health Care Financing Administration has published a summary of the results of five prospective-reimbursement evaluation studies. The studies were conducted on prospective-payment systems of different types in Rhode Island, Western Pennsylvania, New Jersey, upstate New York, and downstate New York. The estimates of savings per hospital day from the programs ranged from 1 percent in upstate New York to 4 percent in downstate New York. When calculated on a per-admission basis, the estimates ranged from 2 percent in upstate New York to 3.1 percent in Rhode Island. However, in many cases, the statistical significance of the estimated impact is low.[31] Sloan and Steinwald concluded that previous research did not indicate that has failed to prospective reimbursement was an effective means for achieving cost containment. Their own research was also consistent with this conclusion.[32]

Coelen and Sullivan have undertaken the most comprehensive empirical study of prospective reimbursement ever completed. Using data from 2,700 community hospitals form 1969–1978, they estimated the effect of prospective-reimbursement programs on hospital expenditures per patient day, per admission, and to a lesser extent, per capita.[33] (See table 4–3).

The statistical evidence indicates that programs in Arizona, Connecticut, Maryland, Massachusetts, Minnesota, New Jersey, New York, and

Table 4–3
Estimated Effects of Prospective Reimbursement Programs on Hospital Cost per Patient Day, per Admission, and per Capita *(Percentage Point Change)*

	Annual Percentage Change			Level of Expenditure		
Program	Expense/ Patient Day	Expense/ Admission	Expense/ Captia	Expense/ Patient Day	Expense/ Admission	Expense/ Capita
Arizona						
Voluntary, 1974–1978		—	—	−4.8	—	—
Connecticut						
Mandatory, 1975–1978	−2.8	−2.6	—	−7.4	−8.7	—
Indiana						
Voluntary, 1969–1978	—	—	—	−6.4	—	—
Kentucky						
Voluntary, 1975–1978	—	—	—	−5.6	—	—
Maryland						
Mandatory, 1976–1978	−6.1	−4.2	—	−5.6	—	—
Massachusetts						
Mandatory, 1976–1978	−3.0	−1.9	−3.1	−5.4	−4.1	—
Minnesota						
Voluntary, 1975–1978	—	—	—	−3.9	−6.5	—
Voluntary, 1978	—	−2.2	—	—	—	—
New Jersey,						
Mandatory, 1977–78	−3.2	−2.7	—	−4.1	—	—
New York						
Mandatory, 1971–1978	−1.2	—	—	−2.7	—	—
Mandatory, 1976–1978	−3.4	−4.6	−4.1	—	—	5.1
Rhode Island						
Mandatory, 1975–1978	—	−4.2	−3.9	—	−8.3	—
Washington						
Mandatory, 1976–1978	—	—	−3.1	—	—	−7.6

Source: Craig Coelen and Daniel Sullivan, "An Analysis of the Effects of Prospective Reimbursement Programs on Hospital Expenditures," *Health Care Financing Review* 2, no. 3 (Winter 1981): 19.

Rhode Island, have reduced the rate of increases from 2 to 6 percentage points. There are no indications of cost reductions for programs in Colorado and Nebraska. There are indications, although less strong, that prospective-reimbursement programs also reduced expenses in Indiana, Kentucky, Washington, Western Pennsylvania, and Wisconsin.

An analysis of the relative effectiveness of the various programs suggests that mandatory programs have a significantly higher probability of influencing hospital behavior than do voluntary programs. Some voluntary programs, however, are shown to be effective.

Only in the most recent years have prospective reimbursement programs been shown to have a statistically and practically significant effect on hospital expenditures.[34] Even the older programs (for example, New York) did not have statistically significant effects until 1975 or 1976. It is not possible to determine at this point whether the lack of any apparent success for early programs was due to the confounding influence of the Economic Stabilization Program or to limitations in program design. The fact that some programs that were implemented in the mid-1970s produced an effect almost immediately does suggest that a program does not have to be in existence for 4 or 5 years before it influences hospital costs.

The study by Coelen and Sullivan, in general, duplicates the empirical results obtained by Sloan and Steinwald in that regulatory variables for the period prior to 1976 (the end of the latter's data series) seldom are statistically significant. However, the implications of the results obtained by Coelen and Sullivan for later years are substantially different. Seven to ten prospective-reimbursement programs in existence after 1975, especially mandatory programs, are shown to be effective in controlling hospital costs.

Certificate of Need

Controls on capital investment and services are fundamental to state and federal efforts for limiting the increase in costs of health care. Three broad types of change are subject to review by appropriate agencies: changes in physical plant (facilities), changes in equipment, and changes in services.

Certificate of need is designed to give government some control over investment in the health sector. To date the approach has been used primarily to limit hospital construction by requiring regulatory approval for projects that exceed a particular dollar amount.

Analysis of the impact of early certificate-of-need programs suggests that this approach has not substantially affected total investment in the hospital sector. Although there has been some reduction in the use of capital to increase bed capacity, investment in new and costly equipment and services has increased. This redirection of investment capital has reduced the utilization of inpatient services by reducing the availability of hospital beds. The net effect, however, has been an increase in the cost of each day of care that is provided.[35]

Moreover existing hospitals are protected to some degree from new competition by the tight restrictions on bed expansion that result from certificate-of-need programs. Because of this, hospitals are able to raise the price of services for all patients, and hospitals can obtain the requisite capital to finance sophisticated new services of sometimes limited usefulness.[36]

A further problem with certificate-of-need programs derives from a failure to define, in many instances, what constitutes an appropriate supply of services. The agencies that administer these programs have no review standards and little information on the utilization of and need for facilities, equipment, and services. Typically the investment plans of one institution are received without information on, or regard for, the plans of other institutions in the area. Lacking useful concepts and operational measures of need, as well as a knowledge of potential investment opportunities, certificate-of-need agencies are unable to select a set of proposals that, when taken together, will produce an optimal pattern of investment.

Summary

Hospital statistics indicate that the average patient's hospital bill totaled nearly $2,142 in 1980, as compared to $127 in 1950. In no other segment of the health-care industry have costs risen so rapidly.

From 1968 to 1979 the most important single factor accounting for increases in hospital expenditures was rises in the prices of hospital inputs. Increases in utilization and intensity of services rendered were of less importance.

Regarding the causes of hospital inflation, the most important single factor appears to be rising demand. The growth of third-party payers, particularly Blue Cross and Medicare, has greatly increased the demand for hospital services.

Several types of reimbursement mechanisms were discussed, with the greatest emphasis focusing on prospective reimbursement. The key factors that determine the way in which prospective reimbursement operates are the payment unit and the rate-setting method.

The empirical evidence indicates that prospective reimbursement has has an increasing effect in containing increases in hospital costs. Apparently, statistically significant effects began to occur after 1975 or 1976. The confounding influence of price controls under the Economic Stabilization Plan may partially account for this result.

Certificate of need is another method, in addition to prospective reimbursement, for cost containment. While there is evidence that certificate-of-need regulations reduced the use of investment for expansion of bed capacity, funds have apparently been redirected toward expensive services and new equipment.

Notes

1. See Karen Davis and Louise Russell, "The Substitution of Hospital Outpatient Care for Inpatient Care," *Review of Economics and Statistics* 54, no. 2 (May 1972): 109–120, for an interesting econometric study of this issue.

2. American Hospital Association, *Hospital Statistics*, 1981 ed. (Chicago: AHA, 1981), p. 191.

3. Ibid., pp. 3–5.

4. Herman Somers and Ann Somers, *Medicare and the Hospitals: Issues and Prospects* (Washington, D.C.: The Brookings Institution, 1967), p. 49.

5. Ibid.

6. Congressional Budget Office, *Controlling Rising Hospital Costs* (Washington, D.C.: U.S. Government Printing Office, 1979), p. ix.

7. Ibid., p. 2.

8. F.A. Sloan and B. Steinwald, *Wage Setting in the Hospital Industry, Evidence from the 60s to 70s*, Final Report, Grant no. HS02590. Prepared for the National Center for Health Services Research, 1979.

9. F.C. Cohen and H.J. Bachofer, "Hospital Indicators," *Hospitals* 54, no. 3 (February 1, 1980): 33–36, 79.

10. Congressional Budget Office, *Controlling Rising Hospital Costs*, p. 4.

11. David Salkever and Alan Sorkin, "Economics, Health Economics, and Health Administration," report prepared for the Association of University Programs in Health Administration, August 1976 (mimeographed), pp. 38–39.

12. Martin Feldstein, *Economic Analysis for Health Service Efficiency* (Chicago: Markham, 1968), pp. 81–86; and M.L. Ingbar and L.D. Taylor, *Hospital Costs in Massachusetts* (Cambridge, Mass.: Harvard University Press, 1968), pp. 148–164.

13. C.A. Watts, W.L. Dowling, and W.C. Richardson, "Strategies for the Reimbursement of Short-Term Hospitals," in Lester Breslow, Jonathan Fielding, and Lester Lave, *Annual Review of Public Health*, vol. I (Palo Alto, Calif.: Annual Reviews, 1980), p. 98.

14. V.P. Goldberg, "Regulation and Administered Contracts," *Bell Journal of Economics* 7, no. 2 (1976): 426–488.

15. Hal Cohen, "Issues in State Rate Regulation," paper presented at Conference on Regulation in the Health Industry, Washington, D.C., 1974 (mimeographed).

16. Ibid.; and R.A. Posner, "Taxation by Regulation," *Bell Journal of Economics* 2 no. 1 (1971): 22–50.

17. Watts, Dowling, and Richardson, "Reimbursement of Short-Term Hospitals," p. 98.

18. Ibid.

19. Salkever and Sorkin, "Economics, Health Economics, and Health Administration," p. 66.

20. W.J. Carr and Paul Feldstein, "The Relationship of Cost to Hospital Size," *Inquiry*, 4, no. 1 (March 1967): 45.

21. J. Holohan, B. Spitz, W. Pollack, and J. Feeder, *Altering Medicaid Provider Reimbursement Methods* (Washington, D.C.: Urban Institute, 1977), p. 39.

22. Watts, Dowling and Richardson, "Reimbursement of Short-Term Hospitals," pp. 105–106.

23. William Dowling, "Prospective Reimbursement of Hospitals," *Inquiry* 11, no.3 (September 1974): 163.

24. Ibid., p. 167.

25. Ibid., p. 169.

26. J.R. Lave, L.B. Lave, and L. Silverman, "A Proposal for Incentive Reimbursement for Hospitals," *Medical Care* 11, no. 2 (1972): 79–90.

27. Salkever and Sorkin, "Economics, Health Economics, and Health Administration," pp. 62–63.

28. R.G. Evans and H. Walker, "Information Theory and the Analysis of Hospital Cost Structure," *Canadian Journal of Economics* 5, no. 3 (August 1972): 398.

29. Joseph Lipscomb, Ira Raskin, and Joseph Eichenholz, "The Use of Marginal Cost Estimates in Hospital Cost-Containment Policy," in Michael Zubkoff, Ira Raskin, and Ruth Hanft, *Hospital Cost Containment: Selected Notes for Future Policy* (New York: Prodist, 1978), pp. 514–537.

30. P. O'Donoghue, *Controlling Hospital Costs: The Revealing Case of Indiana* (Denver, Colo.: Policy Center, 1978), p. 91.

31. Health Care Financing Administration, *Research in Health Care Financing*, HEW Publication no. (SSA)-77-11901 (Washington, D.C.: U.S. Government Printing Office, 1977), pp. 84.

32. Frank Sloan and Bruce Steinwald, "Effects of Regulation on Hospital Costs and Input Use," *The Journal of Law and Economics* 27, no. 1 (April 1980): 107.

33. Craig Coelen and Daniel Sullivan, "An Analysis of the Effects of Prospective Reimbursement Programs on Hospital Expenditures," *Health Care Financing Review* 2, no. 3 (Winter 1981): 1.

34. Ibid., p. 18.

35. David Salkever and Thomas Bice, *Hospital Certificate of Need Controls: Impact on Investment Costs and Use*, American Enterprise Institute, Studies in Health Policy (Washington, D.C.: American Enterprise Institute for Public Policy Research, 1979), p. 73.

36. Ibid., p. 38.

5 The Costs and Benefits of Health Programs

Cost-benefit analysis is a technique used by decision makers to *assist* in choosing among alternative programs or courses of action. The basic steps of cost-benefit analysis always have been used by decision makers, but cost-benefit analysis as a managerial tool was not formalized until 1844, when the Frenchman J. Dupuit wrote a paper on the costs and benefits of alternative public works projects.[1] Since that time cost-benefit analysis has been used extensively to measure the costs and benefits of alternative water projects (irrigation, flood control, hydroelectric power plants), transport projects (road, railways, inland waterways), land-usage projects (urban renewal, recreation), and educational programs. Many of the early cost-benefit studies in the United States analyzed water, transport, and land-usage projects and were conducted by the Army Corps of Engineers in response to the River and Harbor Act of 1927, which requires the corps to determine the costs and benefits of its projects.[2]

Traditionally cost-benefit analysis has been used to determine the desirability of projects where the costs and benefits were readily quantifiable in monetary terms. Only recently has the technique been applied to the selection of projects whose benefits are not readily ascertainable in terms of market prices. For example, to calculate the benefits of a public health program requires that a value be placed on the reduction in pain and suffering and the prolongation of life.

It is much more difficult to quantify in monetary terms the value of an intangible such as health, as in the case of reducing the incidence of cancer or mental illness, than it is to quantify the value of a dam that provides water for irrigation. The dam's value may be measured by the market value of the increased agricultural production, but there is no market for a life saved or a lifetime of mental illness avoided. This does not imply, however, that cost-benefit analysis should not be used in situations where benefits or costs are difficult to quantify. As long as decision makers face the problem of choosing among alternative projects to be funded, these decisions should be made with all available information and by a process that determines the costs and benefits of each project. Consequently the relevant question is not whether the costs and benefits of various projects can be measured precisely. Instead it involves how much weight should be given to cost-benefit analysis in decisions regarding which projects are to be funded.

One theoretical problem with cost-benefit analysis is that it operates from a partial framework and is basically a microeconomics tool. Thus it is assumed that the programs being analyzed will have only a marginal impact on the economic, social, or demographic fabric of society. For example, with regard to health, cost-benefit analysis assumes no changes in prices or quantities of resource inputs or in the pattern of demand for a given set of medical services over time resulting from a particular health or medical-care investment.[3] Moreover, in developing countries the problem of extra-marginal impacts is particularly severe because the incidence and prevalence of infectious and parasitic diseases is so great. If malaria were to be eradicated, there would be major demographic impacts on society, particularly 15–30 years after the health intervention. Without a more sophisticated analytical framework capable of considering such macroeconomic impacts, the public policy decisions based on the results of a microeconomic cost-benefit analysis may be undesirable.[4]

There is general acceptance in economics that a dollar is worth more today than it will be if obtained several years in the future; this is true when the overall price level remains constant. As long as assets are secure, consumers are believed to have a positive time preference, that is, they prefer to consume now rather than in the future. Borrowers are therefore willing to pay interest for the use of capital; and lenders, in a capitalist economy, expect to receive interest. In a socialist economy an accounting or imputed rate of interest is employed to help allocate resources over time.[5] The interest rate that is used to determine the present values of future streams of benefits and future streams of costs is known as the *discount rate*.[6]

Because public projects often yield benefits accruing in the future, these benefits must be discounted by an appropriate interest rate in order to determine their present value. For example, suppose that one is contemplating the construction of a dam. The dam is expected to yield services for a period of 50 years. Let us assume that the annual dollar benefit of the dam is equal to $200,000 per year. The total expected benefits of the dam are equal to

$$\Sigma B = \frac{\$200{,}000}{(1 + r)} + \frac{\$200{,}000}{(1 + r)^2} + \frac{\$200{,}000}{(1 + r)^3} + \frac{\$200{,}000}{(1 + r)^4} + \cdots + \frac{\$200{,}000}{(1 + r)^{50}}.$$

Similarly, if the construction of the dam would take five years at a cost of $3 million per year, the total expected costs would be

$$\Sigma C = \frac{\$3{,}000{,}000}{(1 + r)} + \frac{\$3{,}000{,}000}{(1 + r)^2} + \cdots + \frac{\$3{,}000{,}000}{(1 + r)^5}.$$

The total benefits (ΣB) are then divided by the total cost (ΣC) to obtain the cost-benefit ratio.

Thus the discounting process, which recognizes that a given sum of money to be spent or realized in the future is not worth the same amount as the equivalent dollar value obtained or allocated today, provides a link between present value or cost and expected future benefits or costs.

Special Considerations

A number of special factors must be considered when undertaking a cost-benefit analysis: (1) the effect of inflation, (2) risk and uncertainty, (3) the distribution of benefits, and (4) intangibles.

Inflation can be appropriately handled by either of two methods: either estimate all future benefits and costs in constant prices (that is, simply assume no inflation) or estimate all future costs and benefits in current (that is, inflated) prices, and use as the discount rate an estimate of the private opportunity cost of capital.

One approach to dealing with risky or uncertain outcomes is to adopt some arbitrary cut-off (or pay-back) period. In the case of extremely risky projects, the cut-off period might be as short as 2 or 3 years; in other cases, it might be as long as 30 to 50 years. This method of handling risk or uncertainty would result in the adoption of only those projects capable of generating (discounted) benefits prior to the cut-off that are sufficient to more than cover discounted project costs. This decision rule, which is analagous to the pay-back criteria frequently employed by businessmen in judging the desirability of private investments, implicitly assumes that the risk of uncertainty associated with benefits and costs expected to occur beyond the cutoff date is of sufficient magnitude that the analyst may simply ignore those effects. Extremely short pay-back periods, such as 2 or 3 years, would seldom appear justified in evaluating public projects. Moreover analyses conducted with brief cut-off periods ignore all information regarding subsequent events. Another way of handling the problem of risk and uncertainty is to increase the discount rate applied to benefits and decrease the discount rate applied to costs. This tends to result in a lower ratio of benefits to costs, meaning fewer projects will likely be adopted. This procedure is very arbitrary, however.

A third approach to dealing with uncertainty in a cost-benefit framework is to treat estimated benefits and costs as random variables that can be described by some probability distribution. Suppose, for instance, that an analysis of historical flood patterns suggests that the discounted benefits from a flood-control project will range from 0 (if no flood occurs) to $100 million (if the worst possible flood occurs). In addition, the same analysis would also reveal the probability that floods of intermediate severity would occur. Suppose for illustrative purposes that we can identify only four possible outcomes, as well as the probability of their occurrence:

Value of Discounted Benefits ($ millions)	Probability of Occurrence
0	0.3
30	0.4
50	0.2
100	0.1

The method of determining the expected value of benefits when this type of information is available is as follows:

Expected value of benefits = $(0 \times 0.3) + (\$30 \text{ million} \times 0.4) + (\$50 \text{ million} \times 0.2) + (\$100 \text{ million} \times 0.1) = \$32 \text{ million}$.

The primary difficulty with this method of dealing with uncertainty is the unavailability of the data that are needed in order to determine the necessary probability distributions.

A third issue that the decision maker must consider is the distribution of benefits. Consider the following hypothetical set of public projects for which funding is being contemplated:

Project	B/C Ratio	Gains to Poverty Population
A	8:1	20,000
B	7:1	25,000
C	5:1	29,000
D	2.5:1	32,000
E	1.5:1	34,000

In this hypothetical example, the most efficient project, using cost-benefit criteria, and assuming a fixed budget, is project A, with a cost-benefit ratio of 8:1; but the project with the greatest gain to the poverty population is project E—a project that has the lowest B/C ratio of any of the five projects considered. Given this situation, the analyst must *subjectively* weigh efficiency and distributional considerations. However, an explicit formulation of the information available, will make the alternatives as clear as possible.

A final consideration is the allowance for intangibles. For example, the Ford Foundation conducted a program whose primary objective was to reduce the number of dropouts from the St. Louis public schools. The expected direct benefit of such a program was an increase in the expected lifetime income of high-school graduates in comparison with high-school dropouts. Included among the intangible benefits were improved self-esteem of students, increased social and political consciousness, and a reduction in the incidence of crime and delinquency. Intangible factors are difficult, if not impossible, to quantify, particularly in dollar terms. One of the primary problems with the inclusion or consideration of intangibles is that they are sometimes used to justify inefficient projects.

Cost-Benefit Methodology as Applied to the Health Field

In cost-benefit analysis, as applied to the health field, the total cost of the disease serves as the measure of benefits derived from preventing or eradicating the disease.[7] Costs comprise three elements: (1) loss of production, (2) expenditures for medical care, and (3) the pain, discomfort, and suffering that accompany a disease or illness. Because economists concentrate on measuring the first two elements, the third is often neglected for lack of data and an appropriate methodology.

Expenditures for medical care to treat a disease (or injury) do not constitute the total cost of that disease. The economic costs of illness include two components: direct costs and indirect costs. Direct costs are the expenditures for health services attributable to the disease, such as costs for in-patient care, physicians' fees, and drugs. These expenditures reflect the use of resources. Indirect costs are associated with the loss of output attributable to the disease owing to premature death or disability.

Thus the total (direct plus indirect) costs of a disease serve as a measure of benefits derived from a program that would achieve eradication or control of disease. In a cost-benefit calculation, the comparison is between contemplated additional expenditures for health services and the anticipated reduction in existing costs. This is the essential conceptual framework.

Using information on the direct and indirect costs of illness in 1963 and 1972, Cooper and Rice computed their estimate of the total costs of illness. (See table 5–1).

In 1972 the total cost of illness reached $189 billion (4 percent discount rate). This was more than double the figure for 1963. The major growth from 1963 to 1972 has been in direct costs. Although the addition of the drug

Table 5–1
Total Cost of Illness, 1963 and 1972

	1963		1972	
Cost Component	Amount ($ billions)	Percentage Distribution	Amount ($ billions)	Percentage Distribution
Total	93.5	100.01	188.8	100.0
Direct costs	22.5[a]	24.1	75.2[b]	39.8
Morbidity	21.0	22.5	42.3	22.5
Mortality	49.9	53.4	71.2	37.8

Source: Barbara Cooper and Dorothy Rice, "The Economic Cost of Illness Revisited," *Social Security Bulletin* 39, no. 2 (February 1976): 29.

a. Excludes expenditures for drugs and drug sundries amounting to $4.3 billion.

b. Includes expenditures for drugs and drug sundries amounting to $8.6 billion.

category added $8.6 billion to the 1972 total, even without it direct costs have tripled in the 9 year period. The continually increasing cost of medical care has made direct costs the largest component in the cost of illness, $3.8 billion higher than the costs of premature death. In 1963 mortality costs were about double direct costs. (See table 5–1.)

Of the total cost of illness in 1972 ($189 billion), about $40 billion, or one-fifth, was for persons with diseases of the circulatory system. Accidents cost $27 billion and were followed by diseases of the digestive system and cancer, each costing about $17 billion.[8]

The distribution of costs by diagnosis has also changed slightly from 1963 to 1972. (See table 5–2.)

Diseases of the circulatory system represented about the same share in both years, but accidents have grown in importance because of a relatively higher number of deaths. Neoplasms have dropped with relatively fewer cancer victims in the unable-to-work category.

In 1975 the direct cost of ill health was approximately $119 billion. The cost of morbidity was estimated at $58 billion, and the cost of mortality was about $88 billion.[9] Thus in 1975 the total cost of illness was more than $265 billion, about 17 percent of the GNP. Of that total 55.2 percent was indirect costs and 44.8 percent was direct costs. One recent estimate suggests that about half of the costs of illness are for conditions in which prevention could be useful. If current trends continue, it has been estimated that by the year 2000, direct costs will be $416.4 billion (1975 dollars), and indirect costs will be $176.7 billion.[10]

The foregoing data indicate that direct costs of illness rose from 24.1 percent of total costs in 1963, to 39.8 percent in 1972, and 44.8 percent in 1975. If the estimate for the year 2000 is accurate, over two-thirds of the total cost of illness would be accounted for by direct costs. The primary reason for the increasing proportion of direct cost in relation to total cost is the extraordinarily rapid increase in expenditures for health care.

Table 5–2

Comparison of the Economic Cost of Illness from 1963 and 1972, by Diagnosis

Diagnosis	Amount ($ millions)[a]		Percentage Distribution	
	1963	1972	1963	1972
Total	93,500	188,789	100.0	100.0
Infective and parasitic diseases	2,135	3,443	2.3	1.8
Neoplasms	10,590	17,367	11.3	9.2
Endocrine, nutritional and metabolic diseases	2,623	5,930	2.8	3.1
Diseases of the blood and blood-forming organs	373	921	0.4	0.5
Mental disorders	7,277	13,917	7.8	7.4
Diseases of the nervous system and sense organs	6.795	10,951	7.3	5.8
Diseases of the circulatory system	20,948	40,060	22.4	21.2
Diseases of the respiratory system	7,413	16,454	7.9	8.7
Diseases of the digestive system	7,837	17,487	8.4	9.3
Diseases of the genitourinary system	2,560	6,546	2.7	3.4
Complications of pregnancy, childbirth, and the peurperium	1,517	2,932	1.6	1.6
Diseases of the skin and subcutaneous tissue	450	2,052	0.5	1.1
Diseases of the musculoskeletal system and connective tissue	2,783	8,948	3.0	4.7
Congenital anomalies	1,243	1,903	1.3	1.0
Accidents, poisonings, and violence	11,811	26,678	12.6	14.1
Other	7,146	13,294	7.6	7.0

Source: Barbara Cooper and Dorothy Rice, "Economic Cost of Illness Revisited," *Social Security Bulletin* 39, no. 2 (February 1976): 31.

a. Present value of future earnings is calculated at a 4 percent discount rate.

To calculate the economic loss from premature mortality, the estimated value of all deaths is the product of the number of deaths and the expected value of an individual's future earnings.[11] This method of calculation must consider the changing pattern of earnings at successive ages, varying labor-force participation and unemployment rates, work life expectancy for different age and sex groups, and the appropriate discount rate to convert a stream of costs or benefits into its present value.

In order to estimate rigorously the present value of future losses resulting from morbidity, longitudinal data are required on the pattern of illness by diagnosis. If a particular illness strikes an individual in the early years of his working life, how will this affect his productivity in future years? Some illnesses may totally incapacitate him for part of his life, still others may result in a lifetime of partial disability. Although a person cannot die twice, he can be ill or disabled from the same disease more than once.[12] If longitudinal data relating to morbidity patterns by diagnosis cannot be obtained, the analyst can assess the total economic impact of morbidity from specific illnesses. When longitudinal data are not available (which is generally the case), estimates are made simply by multiplying the individual's annual earnings by the fraction of the year he is not available for productive work. This procedure ignores losses in future earning power associated with the illness, of course.

Methodological Issues

The Discount Rate

As indicated previously, a given amount of money has different values when it is realized or spent at different times. The process of discounting converts a stream of benefits or costs into its present value. The higher the rate of discount, the lower the present value of a future income stream. Discounting is particularly important when a long time span is involved, as in a public program where some benefits may accrue 30 to 50 years after the outlay.

Although economists agree that a discount rate is necessary for determining the level of benefits that accrue and costs that are incurred, they do not agree on the size of the discount rate. Marked differences of opinion occur for a number of reasons. One is that a variety of interest rates prevail in the real world, owing to capital market imperfections, differences in risk, and governmental monetary policies.[13] In addition, there are philosophical differences among economists on this matter: whether the proper measure of the discount rate for public projects is the opportunity cost of capital in the private sector, or, to the contrary, should the discount rate be reflected in the social rate of time preference? The private rate may be high, well above 10 percent, particularly when allowance is made for the corporate income tax of 50 percent.[14] The social rate of time preference is usually much lower, based on a longer time horizon and presumed greater readiness by society at large than by individuals to postpone consumption in favor of future generations.

Most economists use some interest rate between the market return on private investments and the rate at which the government borrows money (the long-term bond rate). Because there is no universally acceptable method of discounting, it seems reasonable that cost-benefit studies should incorporate estimates of costs and benefits using both low and high interest rates rather than attempt to derive an optimal interest rate.[15]

Housewives' Service

The value of housewives' services is recognized, despite the fact that such services are not exchanged in the market and are excluded from the GNP. In an earlier study by Rice,[16] the value of housewives' services was based on the earnings of a domestic servant. Most observers considered this method of valuation resulted in an underestimate of the value of housewives' services. More recently other approaches to the problem have been developed, including the opportunity-cost and market-cost methods of valuation.[17] Briefly the opportunity-cost approach assumes the economic value of unpaid work to be at least as much as the wage rate that the same person would obtain in the marketplace. The wage rate would be a function of age, education, and on-the-job training. In essence, if a woman chooses housework over employment, the housework must be equal to or greater than the value of the employment.[18] One criticism of this method of valuing housewives' services is that it would not be consistent with the approach used for the employed population. In the latter case one's present activity is valued, as opposed to what one could be doing. A physician in research or academic medicine, for example, could earn much more in private practice, yet only his earnings as a researcher or teacher are counted.

The market-value approach assigns a price to each duty a housewife performs. Based on a time-motion study of housewives, the relevant market wages for various services performed are multiplied by the number of hours reported for doing that service.[19] That figure represents an estimate of the cost of hiring employees to replace the housewife in each of her several activities. It takes into consideration the housewife's age, number of children, and age of youngest child. The psychic value of a housewife to her family or society is not considered in this calculation since any estimate of this value would be highly subjective.

Presence of Multiple Diseases

The presence of disease B when intervention is attempted in disease A serves to raise the cost of intervention and therefore the corresponding benefits.[20] The reason that indirect benefits, which represent gains in future earnings, are also affected is that the presence of diseases A and B in a patient may reduce the probability of successful outcome from the treatment of either. The effect is to overstate the benefits expected from reducing the incidence of one or the other disease.[21] The magnitude of this effect is not known.

When a person is experiencing two or more illness conditions at the same time, the direct and indirect costs incurred cannot be ascribed to a single cause. The presence of multiple conditions results in an overstatement of costs ascribed to any particular condition, when the economic costs are measured separately. The degree of overstatement is a function of the magnitude of interrelatedness of the illness conditions. In this situation the total indirect costs cannot be added together to estimate the total cost of illness to society.

Work-life Expectancy

Calculation of indirect benefits is based on the implicit assumption that the life expectancy of potential survivors is known. Usually standard life tables are employed, separately for men and women. As Weisbrod recognized more than two decades ago, survivors who have avoided a particular cause of death may have a higher or lower susceptibility to other competing causes of death.[22] Klarman compared the effects of simply deleting heart disease as a cause of death on life expectancy and on work-life expectancy. The former was large (11 to 12 years) and latter was small (less than 1 year), since the greatest incidence of heart disease occurs when a person is close to retirement age.[23] For a disease with heavier impact at the younger ages, the effect on work-life expectancy would be relatively larger and correspondingly greater attention would have to be paid to the effect of competing causes of death.

Allowance for Consumption

For some years there was controversy in the cost-benefit literature regarding whether or not consumption expenditures should be deducted from expected income in order to determine the net gain to society from a specific health program. The crucial question was whether or not the potential survivor was regarded as a member of society as opposed to being a member of an individual family.[24] If the latter is true, from the societal viewpoint consumption should not be deducted from earnings, and conversely.

At present consumption by survivors is no longer subtracted from gross earnings in order to obtain net future earnings. Viewed prospectively, everybody is a member of society, including the patient. However, one can argue that in developing countries, especially those with severe population pressure, a deduction for consumption should be made because of the acute scarcity of resources. Stephen Enke made this deduction in his work on the costs and benefits of family-planning programs in developing countries.

A deduction for consumption for retired persons gives a negative estimate of the value of their lives in money terms. Some persons have incorrectly interpreted this as implying that these persons should be eliminated in order to raise society's output. This is a rather bizarre interpretation of cost-benefit analysis.

Calculation of Output Loss

The appropriate measure of output loss is year-round, full-time earnings, not income. The latter includes income from property that would continue in the event of sickness and would be received by one's heirs in the event of one's death.

It can be argued that the appropriate measure of output loss is not earnings but output per worker. However, this implies that labor is the only factor of production deserving remuneration (a Marxist notion) and that such factors as land, capital, or entrepreneurship have no productive contribution. Yet in a severe epidemic in which much capital equipment is idle, output per worker may be the more appropriate measure of output loss. In the same vein the production losses from a natural disaster, such as a flood, tornado, or hurricane, would be more accurately estimated on an output-per-worker basis rather than simply calculating lost earnings.

Measurement of Intangibles

Pain, discomfort, and grief are among the indirect costs of illness and constitute the intangible benefits of a program of health services that averts them. The benefits accrue to the individual, as well as his friends, relatives, and perhaps to society at large. The significance of the latter depends on the extent to which persons take pleasure in the happiness of others.

Weisbrod avoided the problem of valuing intangible benefits by assuming proportionality to tangible benefits.[25] This is an unsatisfactory solution, given the differential impacts of various diseases on life expectancy, disability, and morbidity.

Although this aspect of illness cannot be fully taken into account, it is undoubtedly reflected in the allocation of resources. The pain connected with cancer is probably partly responsible for the relativley large appropriation of federal research funds to combat this disease. The federal budget shows cancer receiving about 18 percent of 1975 federal research dollars, even though the disease represents only 9 percent of the total cost of illness (excluding pain and suffering).[26]

Rate of Employment

Economists typically assume a full-employment unemployment rate of four percent. This implies an employment rate of 96 percent. In the 1970s the full-employment unemployment rate rose. However, whatever the magnitude, Mushkin's view is widely accepted that the health-services system should not be charged with failures by the economy to provide jobs to all who seek them.[27]

As indicated previously, the estimate of lifetime earnings takes into account varying labor-force participation rates and unemployment rates at different ages. The assumption is that an individual will be in the labor force and earning income during his expected lifetime following the pattern of his sex and race group. For example, assume that the average earnings of males age 35–44 is $16,000, with a labor-force participation rate of 96 percent and an unemployment rate of 5 percent. Then the expected earnings of a 35-to-44-year-old male is $16,000 × .91 (0.96–0.05) or $14,560. This assumes that the illness has no long-term effect on the individual's productivity.

Examples of Cost-Benefit Studies

A number of studies have been undertaken to evaluate the costs and benefits of research leading to the development of vaccinations for certain illnesses and the costs and benefits of the vaccination programs themselves. Schoenbaum et al. examined the effects of the rubella vaccine within a cost-benefit framework.[28] The benefits of the vaccination program were defined to include the expenditures that would have been made to treat the disease and its complications had it not been prevented, and the avoidance of work loss. The costs considered were the expenditures for the vaccine, administration of the vaccination program, and treatment of complications of vaccination. The cost-benefit ratio for the monovolent rubella vaccine given to 1 million females was found in this study to be 25 to 1.

A number of difficulties in estimating the benefits and costs of rubella vaccinations have been noted. Because the focus of a rubella vaccination program is primarily the unborn fetus, the availability and acceptability of abortion as an alternative to the birth of a child should be considered explicitly in any analysis. Also the assumption that children are the principal source of disease transmission is apparently an unresolved research question.

Another example of a public health prevention strategy is fluoridation of community water supplies to prevent dental caries. In 1975 more than 105 million Americans resided in communities with appropriately fluoridated water supplies.[29] Walsh reports that current costs of water fluoridation range between 10 and 40 cents per capita per year.[30]

A cost-benefit ratio of more than 6 to 1 for community water fluoridation was found in Hastings, New Zealand, after a fluoridation program had been in effect 10 years.[31] An Australian study found that the benefits of making fluoride tablets available from birth to age 6 were seven times the costs.[32] The potential cost-benefit ratio from school water fluoridation in the United States was estimated to be around 15 to 1.[33] The characteristically high cost-benefit ratios indicate that fluoride programs contribute to a reduction in dental expenditures to a degree that far outweigh their costs.

Providing abortion at public expense through the Medicaid program has been quite controversial because it is a moral issue as well as a public health issue; however, the cost-benefit studies concerning abortion have been favorable although somewhat incomplete. For example, Campbell calculated a cost-benefit ratio for abortion for low-income families of 26 to 1, and a ratio for abortion of illegitimate children of 128 to 1.[34] Such studies usually compare the cost of abortion with the cost of raising children but do not include the potential future earnings of the unborn child as an offset to the cost of raising the child. Therefore the benefit-cost ratios calculated by Campbell are somewhat too high.

A more limited approach has been taken by Cutright and Jaffe, who compared the cost of abortion in poor families with the resultant short-term savings (1 or 2 years) in government costs for medical care and public assistance. The cost-benefit ratio of abortion over the period of study (1970–1975) was 1.8 to 1.[35] This evaluation does not consider the economic costs and benefits to the family, but from the government's prospective, the cost to the Medicaid program for abortion are far lower than the costs for medical care during pregnancy and afterward.

Cost-Benefit Analysis in Developing Countries

The information needed to undertake a fairly complete cost-benefit study is extensive. One requires information on earnings by age and sex, labor-force participation and unemployment rates by age and sex, life tables that permit determination of the probability of living to retirement age, statistics on the direct expenditures for health services, as well as data on the distribution of deaths and morbidity by age and sex for the disease or diseases under consideration. Very little of such information is available in developing countries, forcing researchers to make estimates of the magnitude of the parameters involved.

Moreover agricultural and other subsistence-level workers in many developing countries are often not part of the cash economy, although they may occasionally engage in some market transactions. Nevertheless they do engage in production and consumption of commodities, and thus their premature mortality and morbidity has economic consequences. Since much of the labor force in developing countries is engaged in subsistence agriculture, the measurement of the economic cost of disease for this group is a major and important challenge.

Finally there is considerable evidence that chronic unemployment (both open and disguised) exists in many developing countries, especially in the agricultural regions. This may amount to as much as one-fourth of the labor force.[36] To determine the value of lost production due to premature mortality and morbidity given underemployment of this magnitude is an extremely difficult task.

A recent cost-benefit study of measles vaccination was completed in Southern Zambia. The primary costs of the measles vaccination program are the salaries of the health-care workers and their transportation. These vary from $1-$3 per child vaccinated in urban areas, to $7-$10 per child vaccinated in rural areas. The marginal cost of the vaccine itself was only $0.14 per child vaccinated.[37]

Benefits were calculated (from the viewpoint of the government) in terms of savings in the use of health services and gains in economic output. Fees paid by parents to traditional healers (herbalists or witch doctors) may be considerable; but for the calculation of savings to the government, they were irrelevant and therefore were excluded. This is because the government is interested in reducing the number of persons seeking treatment at government health facilities. If this declines because of improved health, the government will be able to economize on the use of health resources.

The ultimate aim of a measles-control program in developing countries is to reduce the high morbidity and mortality rates due to measles. Since mortality rates are high, it seems reasonable to express the costs and benefits in terms of one life *probably* saved. The limitation "probably" is required since a child who is protected from measles might still die later from another cause such as malnutrition. The costs and benefits of measles immunization are presented in table 5-3.

In this particular study benefits exceed costs in the two urban areas included, but costs likely exceed benefit in the rural areas of Southern Zambia. Thus the results indicate that prevention is not always cheaper than treatment; and if measles-immunization programs are carried out in rural

Table 5-3
Costs and Benefits of Measles Immunization in Southern Zambia

Marginal Cost in Namwala District	In Monze Town	In Nawala Town	75% Coverage	100% Coverage
Cost	K19.50–34.20	K41.35–72.30	K102.75–179.85	K307.55–538.20
Ratio to Monze Town	1	2:1	5.2:1	15.75:1

Economic Benefits Compared with Namwala Town in Namwala District	In Monze Town[a]	In Namwala Town	75% Coverage Offered[a]	100% Coverage Offered
Saved treatment costs	A	K 32.95–132	B	C
Avoided loss to economy	K150	K150	K150	K150
Total benefits	A	K138–282	B	C

Source: Adapted from J.M. Ponnighaus, "The Cost-Benefit of Measles Immunization: A Study from Southern Zambia," *Journal of Tropical Medicine and Hygiene* 83, no. 3 (August 1980):145.
a. A = more, B = less, C = much less.

areas, other programs, such as the extension of basic rural health services, may have to be curtailed because of the costs involved with the former.

Criticisms of Cost-Benefit Analyses of Health Programs

There have been objections to the so-called human-capital approach to cost-benefit analysis, which values life in terms of people's expected earnings. This is partly because it assumes that changes in earnings streams bear a direct relationship to what society values in terms of health-program outputs. Because of income differences, men are valued higher than women, whites higher than other races, and those in the prime working ages higher than the very young and very old.[38]

Mishan and Acton contend that maximizing the present value of earnings streams is not the primary goal of health programs and thus the change in earnings streams attributable to a health program should not be used to measure desirability.[39] In addition, programs to assist the poor, such as the Medicaid program, would rate a low priority using cost-benefit analysis, since the expected earnings of low-income persons are not high. Finally the Medicare program would never be justified on the basis of cost-benefit analysis, since the program recipients are retired and for the most part no longer earning income.

Another approach to estimating the value of health output, known as the "willingness to pay," was first proposed in 1968 by Thomas Schelling.[40] It measures the value of human life by surveying persons to determine how much they are willing to pay to achieve a specified reduction in the probability of death or disability.

Suppose, for example, a certain highway-safety program reduces the risk from death on a highway from 1 in 50,000 to 1 in 100,000. If we could determine how much each person would pay to reduce his risk accordingly, and then sum these amounts, we then could measure the benefit of the program by this method.[41]

Such surveys permit the respondents to indicate different relative preferences for various health outcomes concerning a number of health problems, as well as the relative attractiveness of these outcomes in comparison with expenditures for non–health-related goods that could be purchased for the same amount. The major weakness of the approach is the likelihood that the respondents may not fully understand the questions, and considerable uncertainty exists about the validity and consistency of the responses. For example, on a day when you have stomach pains, programs to combat digestive diseases may seem "worth" far more to you than they do on a day when you have a respiratory ailment. There is a further question of how the respondents perceive the differences between a 1 percent reduction in the probability of death and a 0.1 percent reduction. If all payments come from the consumer, the distribution of income must exert a sizable influence; by how much would willingness to pay change if the task of reducing the death rate were viewed as a collective responsibility that is fully financed from public funds? Because of the immature development of this approach, it has not been emphasized in this volume.

Cost-Effectiveness Analysis

Cost-effectiveness analysis differs from cost-benefit analysis in that costs are calculated and alternative ways are compared for achieving *a specific set of results*. The objective is not just how to use funds most efficiently; it also includes the constraint that a specified output must be achieved. This output is not generally expressed in dollars,[42] but in terms of a particular *health objective* such as years of life saved, number of cases of blindness prevented, number of births averted, or number of addicts successfully treated. Cost-benefit studies expedite comparisons among several programs with differing objectives, whereas cost-effectiveness analysis is used in a comparison of differing ways of reaching the same objective.

Cost-effectiveness analysis is a way of summarizing the health benefits and resources used by health programs so that policy makers can choose among them.[43] It summarizes all program costs into one number, all program benefits (effectiveness) into a second number, and it prescribes rules for making decisions based on the relation between the two. The method is particularly useful in the analysis of preventive health programs, because it provides a mechanism for comparing efforts addressed to different diseases and populations.[44] Cost-effectiveness analysis does not attempt to assign monetary values to health outcomes or benefits.

An alternative widely used formulation is that cost-effectiveness analysis is a method to determine which program accomplishes a given objective at minimum cost.

Example of a Cost-Effectiveness Study

Graduate Turkish midwives were trained to utilize triage rules for determining family-planning home-visit frequency based on risk of couples. A simple method was developed for classifying all eligible couples (married with the wife between ages of 15 and 49) into one of three priority groups. Midwives were trained to assign couples to priority groups on the basis of two easily determined risk factors: the probability of having a future pregnancy, and the probability of experiencing a pregnancy-related complication.[45]

The application of these two criteria leads to the assignment of couples into one of three priority groups:

1. First-priority couples are at high risk of an additional pregnancy and at high risk of a pregnancy-related complication.
2. Second-priority couples are at high risk of an additional pregnancy but at low risk of a pregnancy-related complication.
3. Third-priority couples are at low risk of an additional pregnancy and at low risk of a pregnancy-related complication.

The average costs per new family planning adopter are $30 for priority 1 couples, $33 for priority 2 couples, and $43 for priority 3 couples. (See table 5–4.) The comparison suggests that a home-visiting program that focuses on higher-risk subgroups in a target population can be relatively cost-effective in recruiting adopters from higher-risk groups. Unless other benefits could be demonstrated or less costly recruitment techniques developed, home visiting times should be shifted from the lower-risk couples to the higher-risk couples.

Table 5-4

Cost-Effectiveness Information for the Midwife Home-Visiting Program, by Priority Group

Cost-effective Information [a]	Priority Group		
	1	2	3
Cost per adopted (experimental)			
Number of couples in sample	66	245	231
Number of home visits	218	632	471
Number of modern method adopters	6	16	9
Cost per adopter	$30	$33	$43
Cost per complication averted (estimated)			
Estimated fecundity rate	100%	75%	50%
Estimated contraceptive success rate	75%	75%	75%
Estimated pregnancy complication rate	66%	33%	22%
Estimated number of complications averted	2.97	2.97	.74
Estimated cost per complication averted	$61	$177	$526

Source: Adapted from Robert Bertera and Lawrence Green, "Cost-effectiveness of a Home Visiting Triage Program for Family Planning in Turkey," *American Journal of Public Health* 69, no 9 (September 1979): 953.

a. Cost information common to all three priority groups: midwife hourly salary is $1.10; average length of a home visit is 0.75 hours; and the average cost of a home visit is $0.83.

Summary

Cost-benefit analysis has traditionally been used to evaluate projects in the areas of irrigation, flood control, and transportation. More recently the technique has been applied to human-resource-development programs, including health services.

The cost of ill health comprises three elements—direct costs, indirect costs (premature mortality and morbidity), and pain and suffering. In a cost-benefit exercise, a comparison is made between expected program expenditures and the anticipated reduction in the cost of illness (the measure of benefits).

A number of methodological issues must be considered when carrying out a cost-benefit study of a health program. These include the choice of discount rate, the valuation of housewives' services, the presence of multiple diseases, the allowance for consumption, the calculation of output loss, and the measurement of intangibles.

Cost-benefit analysis has been criticized for assuming that variations in expected lifetime income are directly related to what society values in terms of the output of health programs. This results in lower values being assigned, for example, to females and members of minority groups because their incomes are less than white males.

The willingness-to-pay approach to valuing the output of health services does not suffer from the aforementioned weakness but requires a highly sophisticated populace in order to obtain even minimally useful results.

Cost-effectiveness analysis is an alternative way of evaluating health programs. This method determines relevant program costs and compares alternative ways of obtaining a particular set of results. It has the advantage that output is not expressed in dollars. Thus the analyst does not have to deal with the thorny problem of determining the monetary value of human life.

Notes

1. J. Dupuit, "On the Measurement of the Utility of Public Works," in Kenneth Arrow and Tibor Scitovsky (Eds.), *Readings in Welfare Economics* (Homewood, Ill.: Richard D. Irwin, 1969), p. 41.

2. Fred Hellinger, "Cost-Benefit Analysis of Health Care: Past Applications and Future Prospects," *Inquiry* 17, no. 3 (Fall 1980): 204.

3. David Dunlop, "Benefit-Cost Analysis: A Review of Its Applicability in Policy Analysis for Delivering Health Services," *Social Science and Medicine* 9, no. 3 (March 1975): 134.

4. Robin Barlow, *The Economic Effects of Malaria Eradication*, Research Series, no. 15 (Ann Arbor, Mich: University of Michigan, School of Public Health, 1968), p. 13.

5. Herbert Klarman, "Application of Cost-Benefit Analysis to the Health Services and the Special Case of Technologic Innovation," *International Journal of Health Services* 4, no. 2 (1974): 328.

6. Herbert Klarman, *The Economics of Health* (New York: Columbia University Press, 1965), p. 165.

7. Burton Weisbrod, *Economics of Public Health* (Philadelphia, Pa.: University of Pennsylvania Press, 1961), p. 90.

8. Barbara Cooper and Dorothy Rice, "The Economic Cost of Illness Revisited," *Social Security Bulletin* 39, no. 2 (February 1976): 29.

9. A. Berk, L.C. Paringer, and S.J. Mushkin, *The Economic Cost of Illness, 1975* (Washington, D.C.: Georgetown University Public Services Laboratory, 1977), p. 37.

10. S.J. Mushkin et al., "Cost of Disease and Illness in the United States in the Year 2000," *Public Health Reports*, Supplement, vol. 93, no.5 (September-October 1978): 494.

11. Weisbrod, *Economics of Public Health* p. 33.

12. Dorothy Rice, "Estimating the Cost of Illness," *American Journal of Public Health* 57, no. 3 (March 1967): 437.

13. A.R. Prest and R. Turvey, "Cost-Benefit Analysis: A Survey," *Economic Journal* 75, no. 300 (1965): 683–735.

14. W.J. Baumol, "On the Discount Rate for Public Projects," in R.H. Haveman and J. Margolis (Eds.), *Public Expenditures and Policy Analysis* (Chicago: Markham, 1970), pp. 273–290.

15. Hellinger, "Cost-Benefit Analysis of Health Care," p. 207.

16. Rice, "Estimating the Cost of Illness."

17. Wendyce Brody, *Economic Value of a Housewife* Research and Statistics Note no. 9 (Washington, D.C.: Social Security Administration, Office of Research and Statistics, 1975), p. 21.

18. Reuben Gronau, "The Measurement of Output of the Nonmarket Sector: The Evaluation of Housewives' Time," in Milton Moss (Ed.), *The Measurement of Economic and Social Performance* (New York: National Bureau of Economic Research, 1973), pp. 168 and 171.

19. Katherine Walker and William Gauger, "The Dollar Value of Household Work," *Information Bulletin* College of Human Ecology, Cornell University, Ithaca, N.Y., 1973, p. 16.

20. Herbert Klarman, "Syphilis Control Programs," in Robert Dorbman (Ed.), *Measuring Benefits of Government Investments* (Washington, D.C.: The Brookings Institution, 1965), pp. 367–410.

21. Selma Mushkin, "Health as an Investment," *Journal of Political Economy* 70, no. 5 (1962): 129–157.

22. Weisbrod, *Economics of Public Health*, pp. 34–35.

23. Herbert Klarman, "Conference on the Economics of Medical Research," in *Report of the President's Commission on Heart Disease, Cancer, and Stroke*, vol. 2 (Washington, D.C.: U.S. Government Printing Office, 1965), pp. 631–644.

24. E.J. Mishan, "Evaluation of Life and Limb," *Journal of Political Economy* 79, no. 4 (July-August 1971): 690.

25. Weisbrod, *Economics of Public Health* p. 96.

26. Cooper and Rice, "The Economic Cost of Illness Revisited," p. 21.

27. S.J. Mushkin and F. d'A Collings, "Economic Costs of Disease and Injury," *Public Health Reports* 74, no. 9 (1959): 795–809.

28. S.C. Schoenbaum, J.N. Hyde, L. Bartoshesky, and K. Crampton, "Benefit-Cost Analysis of Rubella Vaccination Policy," *New England Journal of Medicine,* 294, no. 4 (February 5, 1976): 306.

29. Richard Scheffler and Lynn Paringer, "A Review of the Economic Evidence on Prevention," *Medical Care* 18, no. 5 (May 1980): 479.

30. D.C. Walsh, "Fluoridation, Slow Diffusion of a Proved Preventive Measure," *New England Journal of Medicine* 296, no. 19 (May 12, 1977): 1118.

31. Scheffer and Paringer, "Economic Evidence on Prevention," p. 479.

32. Ibid.

33. J.P. Carlos (Ed.), *Prevention and Oral Health*, DHEW Publication no. (NIH)74-707 (Washington, D.C.: U.S. Government Printing Office, 1973), p. 25.

34. A.A. Campbell, "The Role of Family Planning in the Reduction of Poverty," *Journal of Marriage and the Family* 30, no. 2 (1968): 236.

35. P. Cutwright and F.S. Jaffe, *Impact of Family Planning Programs on Fertility: The U.S. Experience* (New York: Praeger, 1977), p. 114.

36. N.S. Buchanan and H.S. Ellio, *Approaches to Economic Development* (New York: Twentieth Century Fund, 1955), p. 45.

37. J.M. Ponnighaus, "The Cost-Benefit of Measles Immunization: A Study from Southern Zambia," *Journal of Tropical Medicine and Hygiene* 83, no. 3 (1980): 141–149.

38. Cooper and Rice, "The Economic Cost of Illness Revisited," pp. 27–28.

39. Mishan, "Evaluation of Life and Limb"; and J.P. Acton, *Measuring the Monetary Value of Life-Saving Programs* (Santa Monica, Calif: The Rand Corporation, 1976), p. 82.

40. Thomas Schelling, "The Life You Save May Be Your Own," in S.B. Chase (Ed.), *Problems in Public Expenditure Analysis* (Washington, D.C.: The Brookings Institution, 1965), pp. 142–145.

41. Hellinger, "Cost-Benefit Analysis of Health Care," p. 208.

42. Warren Smith, "Cost-Effectiveness and Cost-Benefit Analyses for Public Health Programs," *Public Health Reports* 83, no. 11 (November 1968): 899–900.

43. Donald Shepard and Mark Thompson, "First Principles of Cost-Effectiveness in Health," *Public Health Reports* 94, no. 6 (November-December 1979): 535.

44. J.R. Lane et al., "Economic Impact of Preventive Medicine," in *Preventive Medicine, U.S.A.* (New York: Prodist, 1976), pp. 675–714.

45. Robert Bertera and Lawrence Green, "Cost-Effectiveness Evaluation of a Home Visiting Triage Program for Family Planning in Turkey," *American Journal of Public Health* 69, no. 9 (September 1979): 950.

6

Health and Economic Development in Developing Countries

To what extent does health accelerate development, and to what degree does development improve health? A substantial amount of research has been devoted to these questions by economists, demographers, and public health specialists during the past 30 years. The purpose of this chapter is to synthesize some of the existing literature in this area, emphasizing the relationship between health and development in poor countries.

Much recent research is based on the framework of human capital theory.[1] In the most general sense human capital is defined as any activity that renders human beings more productive. However, the term is usually used in relation to expenditures on education, health, on-the-job training, or migration. These expenditures are termed investments in human capital. To the extent that better health results in higher income, expenditures made by an individual or a community to improve health status can be considered as resulting in the acquisition of human capital. This investment generates revenues in future years and also may be subject to depreciation. Rates of return or cost-benefit ratios can thus be calculated for health investments in a similar manner to those computed for investments in physical capital.

Once the economic return to particular health programs has been determined, solid information is available for evaluating the policies undertaken by ministries of health and other organizations such as planning agencies, whose activities affect the level of resources devoted to health. Moreover the relative importance of health, in comparison to other social services, can also be considered within the context of this research. Finally knowledge of the interrelationships between better health and rising income is valuable for its own sake.

This chapter will synthesize the literature on health and economic development. Two general impressions will emerge from this summary of the literature. The first is that empirical studies are generally only modestly persuasive. As Ruderman indicates, they are characterized more by anecdotal evidence than by quantitative analysis.[2] Conclusions based on impressionistic findings are widespread. For example, "an intensive [hookworm] control program in the Darjeeling district was *believed* by the manager of a large tea garden to have increased labor efficiency by over 25 percent."[3] When more scientific approaches are used, the research methodology is often weak. The sample size in many studies is too small. Correlations between two variables are often discussed without careful analysis of the direction of causation, or associations between two variables are indicated without an attempt to account for confounding variables or multicollinearity. Variables are represented by proxies that so imperfectly represent the former as to prevent any strong conclusion.

Even when the studies are methodologically sound, it is difficult to draw broad generalizations for them. The research is relevant only within a narrow focus. Consider a study of the effects of a particular disease on the level of per-capita income. The effects in a specific population are likely to be very different from those in some other population. This is because disease-causing agents (such as viruses or parasites) differ in virulence from place to place, and levels of immunity (inherited or acquired) are dissimilar among human populations. The types of treatment for the diseases also differ from place to place and preferences for work as compared to leisure vary from group to group, as do labor market conditions. Thus it is hardly surprising that schistosomiasis is found to be positively associated with absenteeism in one part of the world and negatively in another.[4] The relationships between health and economic development are so complex that definitive studies of many dimensions of this relationship may never be completed.

Before examining specific ways in which health programs impact on economic development, it is necessary to define what economists mean by the "level of development." The single best measure of development is the level of per-capita income. Per-capita income is defined by dividing gross national product by total population. For example, during 1980 the GNP in the United States was $2.632 trillion. The population of the United States in 1980 was 226.5 million, giving a per-capita income of $11,620.

Countries can be ranked, in terms of level of development, by indicating their per-capita income. Nations with per-capita incomes of less than $500 are considered developing nations. Among them are such countries as China, India, Indonesia, Chad, Upper Volta, and Egypt. Nations with per-capita incomes of $500–$2,000 are considered to be in the intermediate stage of development. Examples are Chile, Argentina, South Korea, and a number of countries in Eastern Europe. Nations with per-capita incomes greater than $2,000 are considered to be developed countries. Examples of developed countries are the United States, Canada, Australia, the Soviet Union, and most Western European nations.

One weakness of this approach to development is that it does not consider the *distribution* of income. Two countries with the same per-capita income may have a quite different distribution of income. Since social welfare is to some degree a function of the distribution of income, the country with the more unequal income distribution would be characterized by a lower standard of living for the large mass of the population in comparison to the nation with the more egalitarian income distribution.

The distribution of income is measured by the Lorenz curve. The Lorenz curve shows the cumulative percentage of national income received by cumulative percentages of families.[5] (See table 6–1 and figure 6–1.)

If there were complete equality of income, the Lorenz curve would be a straight line from the origin to the point defined by 100 percent of aggregate income and 100 percent of families. (This is known as the 45 degree line since it bisects the 90 degree angle formed by the intersection of the X and Y axes). With complete inequality of income, the Lorenz curve runs along the horizontal axis and then jumps up to the point defined by 100 percent of the aggregate income and 100 percent of the families.

The closer the Lorenz curve lies to the 45 degree complete-equality line, the greater the equality of the income distribution.

In figure 6–1, the Lorenz curve for Sweden in 1982 is hypothetically drawn to indicate a greater degree of income equality than existed in the United States in that same year. The degree of inequality of income distribution is also reflected in the value of the *Gini index*. The Gini index is the ratio of the area between the Lorenz curve and the complete equality line over the entire area between the complete equality line and the complete inequality line.[6]

The value of the Gini index always lies between 0 (complete equality, with the Lorenz curve on the complete equality line), and 1 (complete inequality, with the Lorenz curve on the complete inequality line). The values of the Gini index show little change has occurred in the distribution of monetary income in the United States from 1947–1976. (See table 6–2.)

Although there are exceptions, as a general rule nations that are less developed (in terms of per-capita income) have more inequality in the

Table 6–1
Percentage Distribution of Income

Percentage of Families	Aggregate Income Received (%)		
	Complete Equality	Complete Inequality	United States 1976
20	20	0	5.4
40	40	0	17.2
60	60	0	34.8
80	80	0	58.9
100	100	100	100.0

Source: U.S. Department of Labor, *Handbook of Labor Statistics, 1977* (Washington, D.C.: U.S. Government Printing Office, 1977), p. 33.

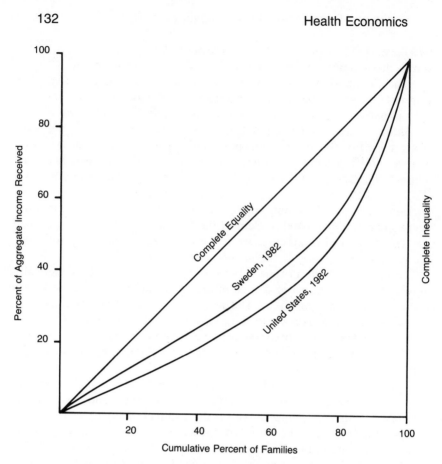

Figure 6-1. Hypothetical Lorenz Curves

distribution of income than nations that are more developed. (See table 6-3.)

Health Programs and Economic Development

There are basically four ways in which health programs can increase the rate of economic development. These are (1) by increasing the potential man hours of productive work, (2) by raising the quality or productivity of the labor force, (3) by opening up new regions of a nation for settlement and development, and (4) by changing attitudes toward innovation and technical progress.

Table 6–2
Gini Index, United States, 1947–1976

Year	Gini Index
1947	.377
1950	.362
1953	.365
1956	.357
1959	.362
1962	.363
1965	.350
1968	.350
1971	.358
1974	.358
1976	.359

Source: U.S. Department of Commerce, Bureau of the Census, *Money Income in 1976 of Persons and Families in the United States*, Current Population Reports P-60, no. 114 (Washington, D.C.: U.S. Government Printing Office, 1978), p. 14.

Table 6–3
Distribution of Income, Selected Countries

Country	Per-Capita Income	Percentage Share of Household Income, by Percentile Groups of Households					
		Lowest 20%	Second Quintile	Third Quintile	Fourth Quintile	Highest 20%	Highest 10%
United States	$9,590	4.5	10.7	17.3	24.7	42.8	26.6
West Germany	9,580	6.5	10.3	15.0	22.0	46.2	30.3
Netherlands	8,410	6.5	11.6	16.4	22.7	42.9	27.7
France	8,260	4.3	9.8	16.3	22.7	46.9	30.4
United Kingdom	5,030	6.3	12.6	18.4	23.9	38.8	23.5
India	180	6.7	10.5	14.3	19.6	48.9	35.2
Honduras	480	2.3	5.0	8.0	16.9	67.8	50.0
Philippines	510	3.7	8.2	13.2	21.0	53.9	——
Peru	740	1.9	5.1	11.0	21.0	61.0	42.9
Malaysia	1,090	3.3	7.3	12.2	20.7	56.6	39.6
Mexico	1,290	2.9	7.0	12.0	20.4	57.7	40.6
Costa Rica	1,540	3.3	8.7	13.3	19.9	54.8	39.5

Source: World Bank, *World Development Report, 1980* (Washington, D.C.: World Bank, 1980), pp. 110–111 and 156–157.

Partly because of the widespread implementation of low-cost health and sanitation programs, death rates have fallen very rapidly in developing countries. In the late 1940s death rates in developing countries averaged 29 per 1,000 population. This figure fell to 19 by 1960, 15 by 1970, and 12 by 1980.[7] Crude birthrates over the same time period fell more slowly from 41 to 33 per 1,000 persons. As a result population and labor force have increased rapidly in the developing world. This increase in potential hours of productive work could result in increased output if jobs were available for these additional workers or if their employment ameliorated a labor shortage.

However, except for a few countries in the Middle East, as well as Switzerland or Japan, where unemployment rates are low, the chief manpower problem is a surplus of labor. In the United States, Canada, and much of Western Europe, unemployment rates range from 10 to 15 percent. In developing countries measured unemployment rates are at least this high and there is the additional phenomenon of disguised unemployment, in which workers (primarily agricultural) have jobs that in reality contribute little or nothing to total output. In some developing countries disguised unemployment may amount to 15–25 percent of the total labor force.

Given this reality, adding more persons to the labor force (or potential labor force) by reducing death rates via health or disease-control programs may fail to increase economic growth but will likely make the unemployment problem worse. This does not mean that for humanitarian reasons these health or disease-control programs should not be undertaken but that they may not also be justified on economic grounds.

Health or nutrition programs may increase the efficiency or productivity of the labor force. The productivity of workers is usually measured in terms of output per man hour.

The positive effect of better health or nutrition on productivity may occur in a variety of ways. The most intuitive is an increase in output made possible by greater physical strength. Moreover nutritional gains among small children may have permanent positive effects on mental ability.

Another factor leading to productivity increases is the reduction in the labor turnover made possible by health improvements. When poor health leads to frequent absenteeism and a high degree of personnel turnover, output is likely to decline, as experienced workers continually become ill and are temporarily or permanently replaced by less experienced workers.[8]

However, the supply of labor is a consequence of economic behavior (reflecting the labor/leisure choice), not a pure consequence of physiological condition. Thus one cannot accept the proposition that better health or nutrition leads to higher productivity as automatically valid.

According to standard utility analysis, the individual supply of labor (market-work time) depends upon (1) the utility of income, decreasing on the margin; (2) the disutility of work, increasing on the margin due to (a) disutility experienced from participating in the work process itself and (b) the opportunity cost of forgone nonwork time.[9] Presumably, health status influences the relevant utility/disutility functions and consequently the healthier individual will have more effective time for both market and nonmarket activities—but the conventional labor-supply analysis does not contain enough information to predict a priori the impact of improved health status on the supply of labor. Its actual effect becomes an empirical question.

A number of studies of the economic effects of poor health have focused on the productivity loss due to schistosomiasis. (See table 6–4.) These data indicate considerable disparity in terms of results. The studies done from 1949 to 1963 were not well designed as judged by the criteria of modern research methodology and did not employ control groups. Moreover, the productivity figure for China is apparently only an impressionistic estimate.

The two most sophisticated studies in terms of experimental design and the utilization of control groups were the studies undertaken on the island of St. Lucia and in Northeast Brazil. In the former productivity was measured in terms of the fertility of women, educational achievement of schoolchildren, and the daily output of workers on a banana plantation. As indicated in table 6–4, there was no evidence that productivity losses occurred (in terms of each of the three productivity measures) among those judged to be clinically ill with the disease. Some observers have criticized the

Table 6–4
Estimated Productivity Loss Due to Schistosomiasis, Various Countries

Author	Country	Productivity Loss (%)
Khalil 1949	Egypt	35
Wright 1951	Egypt	33
Ansari 1955	Egypt	4 to 20
Farooq 1963	Philippines	35
Foster 1967	Tanzania	0–3
Weisbrod 1971	St. Lucia	0
Cheng 1971	China	40
Barbosa and Pererra da Costa 1980	Brazil (northeast)	35

Source: M. Farooq, "Medical and Economic Importance of Schistosomiasis," *Journal of Tropical Medicine and Hygiene* 67, no. 5 (May 1964): 109; R. Foster, "Schistosomiasis on an Irrigated Estate in East Africa—III. Effects of Asymptomatic Infection on Health and Industrial Efficiency," *Journal of Tropical Medicine and Hygiene* 70, no. 8 (August 1967): 185–195; Burton A. Weisbrod et al., *Disease and Economic Development* (Madison: University of Wisconsin Press, 1973), p. 81; T.H. Cheng, "Schistosomiasis in Mainland China: A Review of Research and Control Programs Since 1949," *American Journal of Tropical Medicine and Hygiene* 20, no. 1 (January 1971): 26–53; F.S. Barbosa and D.P. Pererra da Costa, "Incapacitating Effects of Schistosomiasis Mansoni on the Productivity of Cane Cutters in Northeastern Brazil," *American Journal of Epidemiology* 114, no. 1 (July 1981): 102.

authors of this study for undertaking research in a location where the disease was relatively mild. Moreover those children and workers who were too sick to attend school or report for work were not included in the study, thus biasing the results.

The work done by Barbosa and Pererra da Costa in northeast Brazil represents the only sophisticated study that indicates that schistosomiasis has a substantial effect on worker productivity. Clearly the location of the study site has an important effect in terms of results.

Another disease that is highly endemic in the developing world is malaria. Nonetheless, there has been surprisingly little substantive research in terms of the loss in labor productivity due to malaria. One study, reported by Winslow, claimed that antimalaria measures on a Malayan rubber estate resulted in a seventeenfold increase in output per worker.[10]

Mushkin attempted to determine the loss in GNP due to malaria in a hypothetical developing country. She assumed that 80 percent of the population was affected by malaria and that the productivity of the agricultural work force would be reduced by 30 percent during a 3-month period of maximum incidence. However, this was merely an assumption and is, therefore, not based on an empirical study.[11]

The most careful investigation of the impact of malaria on economic development was carried out by Gladys Conly in a newly settled region of Eastern Paraguay. Families were divided into three categories: those with mild malaria, moderate malaria, and severe malaria; and comparisons were made in terms of crop yields, amount of work postponed, and acreage devoted to specific crops. For the families afflicted with severe malaria, aggregate output averaged only 74.5 percent of potential output. Moreover the impact of malaria caused substantial disruption to the families' work effort.[12] Young men abandoned the area despite the abundance of excellent farmland. An effort was made on the farms to offset the effects of illness on the principal cash crops by devoting a larger proportion of available labor to them at the expense of those that were less labor intensive, less demanding in terms of the timeliness of attention, or of less importance to the family. Thus tobacco and cotton were given priority over corn, corn over manioc, and manioc over the small subsidiary crops. The results of this study must be interpreted cautiously because of the limited number of families included in the study sample.

Several studies have attempted to determine the effect of nutritional programs on labor productivity. In Costa Rica it was claimed that by improving the workers' diet, rapid increases occurred in the cubic meters of stone moved per construction worker. From 1943 to 1946 the amount of stone moved per worker increased four times.[13] Similarly the local work force of the Pan American Highway was reported to have increased its rate of concrete paving by three times after the introduction of well-balanced daily meals. However, no control groups were established and these early studies lack the rigorous experimental design of later work.[14]

A recent investigation of rubber workers in Indonesia found that 85 percent of the study group suffered from hookworm infestation. This was largely responsible for the finding that 45 percent of the adult male laborers suffered from iron deficiency anemia. It was found that the productivity of nonanemic laborers was approximately 20 percent greater than the productivity of anemic laborers. Treatment was elemental iron for a period of 60 days (at a cost of U.S.$0.0013 per laborer per day), and this resulted in an increase in productivity of approximately 15 percent for tappers and 20 percent for weeders as compared to control groups.[15]

In Indonesia it would cost approximately U.S.$0.50 per year per person to cure the anemia, and U.S.$0.75 per year per person to reduce hookworm infestation in a given area, including distribution costs. The cost-benefit ratio in terms of latex production alone could be 260:1. (This assumes that additional latex could be sold at existing prices.)

While improvements in health or nutrition status have been found in some cases to reduce absenteeism and increase output per hour of labor, this result may be a mixed blessing. This is because unless output expands, the firms employing these workers would need a smaller labor force in order to produce the same or perhaps even a slightly larger level of output. For example, after malaria control programs were undertaken in the Philippines, it was found that only 75 to 80 percent of the number of laborers were needed to accomplish a given task in comparison with manpower requirements before control measures were undertaken.[16]

Factors that are important in permitting an increase in product output in response to health or nutritionally related productivity increases are appropriate transportation facilities, a product with a sufficiently large price elasticity of demand that revenue expands when price declines, and a sufficient supply of other factors of production such as capital equipment that no production bottlenecks occur.

A third way in which health programs can increase the pace of economic development is by opening up new regions for settlement and development through the control of endemic disease. For example, in the Tuinplaats area of the Republic of South Africa, after malaria was controlled, total production increased 400 percent and the population in the region increased about 120 percent in 11 years.[17] Similarly, in the Rico Doce Valley in Brazil, improvements in transportation and the control of malaria resulted in a rapid increase in economic growth. In 1940 the population of the principal town in the valley was 4,791; by 1950 it was 13,149; and in 1960 it was in excess of 80,000. This resulted, to a considerable degree, from malaria control, the economic impact of excellent transportation facilities, new discoveries of ore, immigration of people from drought areas of the northeast, and the inflow of capital from other sections of Brazil.[18] Similar results have been reported in relation to malaria eradication in the Rapti Valley in the Terai of Nepal, the Awash River Valley in Ethiopia, and more generally in Ceylon (Sri Lanka), Sardinia, and Mexico.

Moreover there is also evidence that the spread of a disease into an area has led to depopulation and a decline in output. This is documented by Hunter with respect to onchocerciasis in Ghana[19] and was also discussed with respect to malaria in Eastern Paraguay. In the latter case the government provided land and tools in order to encourage resettlement from parts of rural Paraguay that were relatively overpopulated. However, no sooner were people settled in the region than they began leaving because of the high incidence of malaria. Some cooperation between economic planners and health planners could have resulted in a combined program that would have resulted in a healthy employed population exploiting the soil and natural resources of a previously underdeveloped area.

One problem in analyzing the impact of disease control on regional development is to determine how much growth is due to the health program itself in comparison to other factors such as improvement in the infrastructure. Although in some cases the health program was required before any economic growth could occur, it is an exaggeration to attribute *all* subsequent growth to the health program.

The reallocation of resources encouraged by health improvements has led to some net increase in output, but the effect is probably less than generally believed. It is not adequately recognized that the output increase occurring in the region with the health improvement is obtained to some degree at the cost of reduced output elsewhere, namely in those other regions from which labor and capital migrate. The economic gain that should be attributed to health improvements is the *net increase* in output from all regions combined, not simply the increase taking place in the region where the health improvement occurred.[20]

A fourth way in which health programs can increase the rate of economic development is through changes in attitudes toward innovation and new ideas. Thus even though available technical innovations could increase the output available from additional labor, the existence of endemic disease may itself reduce energy and bring about a mental state that impedes the acceptance of innovation and change. Indeed one can maintain that it is in matters of attitude that ill health has its greatest negative effect on productivity, particularly in the long run.

Wilfred Malenbaum has recently addressed this issues. He notes that one essential ingredient in any consideration of value of health is the importance of the mental and attitudinal aspects of generating output from inputs in the health field. Specifically the introduction of health service in poor areas significantly affects the attitudes of the population and also is important in terms of increasing both people's life span and energy level.[21]

The deteriorated health status of the farmers in poor areas may consititute a major impediment to the adoption and implementation of readily available improvements in technology. This is partly a matter of physical strength, in that sick persons lack sufficient energy for both the day-to-day discharge of the traditional tasks and the investment of labor necessary for improved technology. Moreover, sick persons are unlikely to devote the attention necessary for forward planning and are more likely to be unwilling to assume the risks associated with new types of production methods.[22]

Malenbaum tested these propositions on the basis of macroeconomic (countrywide) data for twenty-two poor countries. Agricultural output was employed as the dependent variable, with various health, economic, and social measures serving as independent variables.

Using a stepwise regression equation, Malenbaum obtained the following results from the aggregate data:

$$X_1 = 133 + 0.34\,X_2 + 0.038\,X_3 - 0.13\,X_4 - 0.00095\,X_5 - 0.024\,X_6,$$

where X_1 refers to agricultural output; X_2 agricultural labor; X_3 commercial fertilizer; X_4 infant mortality; X_5 the physician-population ratio; and X_6 illiteracy.

The five independent variables account for over 62 percent of all the variation in output between countries. Of the total variation explained, about one-fifth comes from the agricultural variables and almost four-fifths from the health variables; less than 2 percent comes from the degree of literacy.[23]

The data for the developing areas as national units do provide evidence of statistically significant relationships between production and health. Moreover the influence of health factors on output appears to be much larger in comparison with the importance of other variables including agricultural inputs. The degree of intercorrelation among the independent variables is small.

Malenbaum's results are not altogether convincing. For one thing the direction of causation between health and output may be the opposite of what he concludes. Rather than better health raising productivity, it may be that the countries with higher productivity have the means to bring about better health. Furthermore the dating of the variables is inappropriate. Malenbaum explains the change in output during the time period by the level of the health variables at some unspecified time during the period. The findings would be more persuasive if the *change* in productivity were related to the *change* in the health variables. Finally some of Malenbaum's health measures are inputs while others are outputs. Thus the regression equations are not correctly specified. As a result one cannot determine which health variables have a major impact on productivity via attitude change.

The Effect of Development on Disease—Some Negative Consequences

Higher incomes usually lead to increases in certain kinds of consumption that are deleterious to health, such as tobacco, alcohol, and fatty foods. Economic development is normally associated with a decline in the proportion of the labor force employed in occupations requiring considerable manual labor and an increase in the percentage of workers employed in sedentary positions. There is a general decline in physical exercise, which in combination with high-calorie diets produces more frequent obesity and associated cardiovascular disease. Higher incomes are usually associated with industrialization, which often produces health-threatening levels of air and water pollution, as well as creating new occupational hazards to which workers are subjected. The building of highways increases the number of traffic accidents, a major cause of death and injury in many countries. Moreover roads may function as a mechanism for transmission of disease. Although their purpose is to encourage movement of people and goods, these facilities encourage the spread of several kinds of insect-borne diseases. For example, with the expanding road and physical communication networks in Africa, which facilitate population movement, the risk of rapid reinvasion of areas by tsetse (and consequent reinfection) are great. This implies that a policy of strict vigilance and control would be of great practical benefit but would require intercountry cooperation.

Some economic development projects have ecological consequences that are harmful to health. Some of the best-known examples concern the spread of schistosomiasis in areas where land-reclamation projects have expanded the habitat of the water snail, which acts as an intermediate host in the transmission of the disease.[24]

The latter situation illustrates the importance of cooperation between health planners and development planners. Suppose that an irrigation system were being built that would yield benefits (in terms of increased agricultural income) for a period of years. The sum of the benefits of the irrigation system can be expressed as follows:

$$\Sigma B = \frac{B_1}{(1 + r)} + \frac{B_2}{(1 + r)^2} + \frac{B_3}{(1 + r)^3} \cdots \frac{B_n}{(1 + r)^n},$$

where B = benefits and r = discount rate. The cost of the project can be expressed as follows:

$$\Sigma C = \frac{C_1}{(1 + r)} + \frac{C_2}{(1 + r)^2} + \frac{C_3}{(1 + r)^3} \cdots \frac{C_n}{(1 + r)^n}$$

However, since the irrigation project is hypothesized to increase the prevalence of schistosomiasis, this must be considered in computing the *net benefits* of the irrigation project. The cost of illness is generally considered to be the sum of direct or treatment costs, morbidity, and premature mortality. (See chapter 5). These costs must be subtracted from the benefits (increased agricultural income) in order to obtain the net benefits. The following equation expresses this consideration:

$$\Sigma B_n = \frac{B_1 - d_1}{(1 + r)} + \frac{B_2 - d_2}{(1 + r)^2} + \frac{B_3 - d_3}{(1 + r)^3} \cdots \frac{B_n - d_n}{(1 + r)^n},$$

where B = net benefits and d represents the cost of illness. Depending on the illness costs associated with the irrigation project, the planners may decide to continue with the project or to cancel it. Without information from the Ministry of Health on the cost of illness and expected incidence, the benefits of this project would likely be overestimated.

Summary

The level of economic development of a nation is usually measured in terms of per-capita income. The distribution of income is also important in assessing the standard of living for the vast majority of the population. As a general rule the poorer nations of the world have a more unequal income distribution in comparison to the more affluent nations.

Health programs can affect development in four ways: (1) by increasing the number of *potential* man hours of productive work, (2) by raising the efficiency or productivity of the work force, (3) by providing the catalyst for regional development, and (4) by encouraging positive attitudes toward innovation and change.

Because so many nations suffer from an unemployment problem at the present time, health programs or disease-control programs could, in certain situations, make such problems worse. However, disease-control programs that permit previously unsettled regions to be populated and developed will cause both output and employment to increase.

Development programs, under certain circumstances, can have negative impacts on the health status of the population. This possibility should be reflected in cost-benefit studies of development projects. Such work requires collaboration between health planners and development planners.

Notes

1. Robin Barlow, "Health and Economic Development: A Theoretical and Empirical Review," *Research in Human Capital and Development*, 1 (1979): 46.

2. Peter Ruderman, "Introduction to the Theme: Health and Socio-Economic Development," *International Journal of Health Services* 1, no. 3 (1971): 189–192.

3. C.E.A. Winslow, *The Cost of Sickness and the Price of Health* WHO Monograph Series, no. 7 (Geneva, Switzerland: World Health Organization, 1951), p. 19.

4. R. Foster, "Schistosomiasis on an Irrigated Estate in East Africa—III. Effects on Asymptomatic Infection on Health and Industrial Efficiency," *Journal of Tropical Medicine and Hygiene* 70, no. 8 (August 1967): 185–195; and Burton Weisbrod et al., *Disease and Economic Development* (Madison: University of Wisconsin Press, 1973), pp. 22 and 75.

5. Michael Bradley, *Micro-Economics* (Glenview, Illinois: Scott Foresman, 1980), p. 367.

6. Bradley, *Micro-Economics*, p. 368.

7. World Bank, *World Development Report, 1980* (Washington, D.C.: World Bank, 1980), p. 64.

8. Barlow, "Health and Economic Development," p. 57.

9. Carl Stevens, "Health and Economic Development: Longer-Run View," *Social Science and Medicine* 11, no. 17/18 (1977): 810.

10. Winslow, *The Cost of Sickness*, p. 26.

11. Carl E. Taylor and Marie-Francoise Hall, "Health, Population, and Economic Development," *Science* 157, no. 3789 (August 11, 1967): 651.

12. Gladys Conly, *The Impact of Malaria on Economic Development: A Case Study* (Washington D.C.: Pan American Health Organization, 1975), p. 93.

13. Harry T. Oshima, "Food Consumption, Nutrition, and Economic Development in Asian Countries," *Economic Development and Cultural Change* 15, no. 4 (July 1967): 391.

14. Winslow, *The Cost of Sickness*, p.33.

15. S.S. Basta and A. Churchill, "Iron Deficiency Anemia and the Productivity of Adult Males in Indonesia," International Bank for Reconstruction and Development, Staff Working Paper no. 175, April, 1974, p. 1.

16. U.S. Department of Health, Education, and Welfare, Public Health Service, *Report of Philippine Public Health Rehabilitation Program, July 4, 1946–June 30, 1950* (Washington, D.C.: U.S. Government Printing Office, 1950), p. 5.

17. Winslow, *The Cost of Sickness*, p. 25.

18. Mark Perlman, "Some Economic Aspects of Public Health Programs in Underdeveloped Areas," in Bureau of Public Health Economics, *The Economics of Health and Medical Care: Proceedings of the Conference on the Economics of Health and Medical Care, May 10–12, 1962* (Ann Arbor: University of Michigan, 1964), p. 293.

19. John Hunter, "River Blindness in Nangodi, Northern Ghana: A Hypothesis of Cyclical Advance and Retreat," *The Geographical Review* 56, no. 3 (July 1966): 409–410.

20. Barlow, "Health and Economic Development," pp. 58–59.

21. Wilfred Malenbaum, "Health and Economic Expansion in Poor Lands," *International Journal of Health Services* 3, no. 2 (1973): 169.

22. Stevens, "Health and Economic Development," p. 813.

23. Wilfred Malenbaum, "Health and Productivity in Poor Areas," in Herbert Klarman (Ed.), *Empirical Studies in Health Economics* (Baltimore, Md.: Johns Hopkins Press, 1970), p. 38.

24. Barlow, "Health and Economic Development," p. 62.

7

Population Growth and Economic Development

A variety of analytical methods and approaches are employed by economists and demographers to consider the various interrelationships between population growth and economic development. These include macroeconomic analysis, microeconomic analysis, the concept of human capital, the theory of demographic transition, and the role of income distribution in explaining changes in birthrates and rates of population growth. Before considering these issues, it is important to focus on basic factual information regarding world population growth.

Demographic Trends and Projections

Table 7–1 compares past and projected trends in birthrates and death rates in developed and developing countries. Two points need to be emphasized. One is the rapid population growth in the developing world, particularly after death rates declined in the post–World War II years, and the continued rapid growth projected for the rest of this century. The second is the drop in birthrates, which began in the 1960s in the developing world and the resulting gradual slowdown in the population growth rate since then—from a peak of about 2.4 percent in 1965, to 2.2 percent at the present time.

From 1965 to 1980 birthrate declines of at least 10 percent occurred in the world's two most populated countries, China and India, and in a number of other major developing countries—Indonesia, the Philippines, Thailand, Turkey, and South Korea.[1] Moreover the recent rate of decline has been faster in the developing world than it was in the nineteenth-century in Europe and the United States (the period of demographic transition in the developed countries). England and the Netherlands took about 50 years to reduce their birthrates from 35 to 20 per 1,000—or about one point every 3 years; Indonesia, Colombia, and Chile have recently cut about one point every year from their crude birthrates—though generally from higher initial starting points.

Higher incomes, a more equitable distribution of education, and the growing acceptability of family planning programs have begun to reduce birthrates in most middle-income countries in Latin American and East Asia, and in some countries and regions of South and Southeast Asia. Given continued socioeconomic progress, the fertility decline is projected to spread to the rest of South Asia and, with some delay, to Africa, during the 1980s and 1990s.

Even with these fertility declines, world population will continue to grow, however. By 2000 World Bank projections indicate world population will have risen from the current estimate of 4.4 billion in 1980 to about 6 billion. (See table 7−2.) The population of the developing countries (including China) is projected to increase from 3.3 to 4.9 billion. India is projected to grow from 672 to 974 million people; Brazil from 126 to 201 million; Nigeria from 85 to 153 million. These assumptions are based on the assump-

Table 7−1
Trends in Birthrates and Death Rates, 1775−2050

	Developed Countries		Developing Countries	
Year	Crude Birthrate	Crude Death Rate	Crude Birthrate	Crude Death Rate
1775	39	33	42	38
1800	39	32	42	37
1850	39	30	42	37
1900	32	23	42	34
1950	23	11	42	24
1965	19	9	39	18
1975	18	9	37.5	12
1990[a]	17	10	30	9
2000[a]	17	10	28	9
2025[a]	17	11	20	9
2050[a]	17	12	16	10

Source: The World Bank, *World Development Report, 1980* (New York: Oxford University Press, 1980), p. 64.
[a] Projected.

Table 7−2
Current Population Levels and Population Projections for Groups of Countries Classified by Stage of Type of Development *(millions)*

Country Grouping	Population		Hypothetical Size of Stationary Population
	1980	2000	
Low income	1,348	2,050	4,074
Middle income	916	1,409	2,599
Industrialized	673	736	774
Capital surplus oil exporters	64	104	203
Centrally planned economics	1,386	1,730	2,121
Total	4,387	6,029	9,771

Source: World Bank, *World Development Report, 1980* (New York: Oxford University Press, 1980), pp. 142−143.

tion that current rates of social and economic progress, including the spread of family planning and health and education services, will continue.

It is instructive to consider the consequences of an acceleration of fertility decline such as to cause the rate of population growth in particular countries to fall to zero 10 years earlier than currently projected. The size of the resulting stationary populations would be reduced by, for example, 200 million in India, 50 million in Nigeria, and 36 million in Mexico.

Even though declines in the present high birthrates have begun in a number of countries, the age structure remains sharply pyramidal. Therefore a great deal of additional population growth will take place before ultimate stabilization occurs.

Using a standard, plausible, assumption about the rate of future declines in mortality rates and various assumptions regarding the decline in fertility rates to replacement levels, Frejka made projections of worldwide population growth and for the developed and less developed regions separately. The alternative projections of fertility trends assume linear declines in the net reproduction rate to replacement level in periods of 0, 10, 30, 50, and 70 years. The results are of great importance. For the developed countries, the difference between the fastest and slowest fertility decline in terms of total population is only 125 million people by the year 2000 and 525 million by the year 2100. For the less developed countries, the difference by the year 2000 is 2,729 million. This is over 20 times as large as the difference made by the same alternative fertility assumptions for the developed countries. For the year 2100, the difference between the most optimistic and pessimistic assumptions, in terms of population, is 9,612 million.[2] According to Frejka: "One implication of the above findings cannot be stressed enough: long-term population growth of LDCs depends heavily on fertility changes of the near future. This is so because current high fertility is producing large stocks of future child bearers."[3]

In the developed countries fertility is already so low as to be near replacement levels and is unlikely to decline very much in the future.[4] Moreover it is highly likely that income growth in the developed countries will have little net impact on their birthrates. The primary reason for this is that within the developed countries, almost all subgroups have converged to a similar pattern of low fertility. Modern attitudes, contraceptive knowledge, and the opportunities and constraints of modern life are already sufficiently widespread so that a large proportion of households in the developed countries have been affected and have lowered their fertility accordingly.[5]

This is evident in the narrowing of fertility differentials in the developed countries since World War II. Fertility differentials, which were substantial in the nineteenth and twentieth centuries, have narrowed greatly, and, in fact, largely disappeared since 1945. In Europe various differentials had narrowed or become erratic as early as 1960. By 1970 the had converged to such a degree that a leading European demographer could write as follows:

> Over the past century fertility in Western Europe has been steadily declining, and seems to be converging within a fairly slender bracket of between 2.3 and 2.7 births per woman among the generation reaching the reproductive age immediately after the war, declining still further in the most recent further generations. The situation appears to be growing more homogenous, in terms of space, time, and the social hierarchy, as though the family were approaching a model, standard pattern. . . . Differences among countries, regions, and social classes have lessened to such an extent that it seems useless to discuss them unless we wish to split hairs.[6]

The Microeconomics of Population Control

One way to determine the benefits of a birth-prevention program is to estimate the production and consumption streams of an individual at birth. In making this calculation, one is using the concept of human capital to estimate the monetary value of human life.

Assume that per-capita income in a particular country is $100. Suppose that the saving rate is $S = 0.10$ (meaning that 10 percent of income is saved), and the appropriate discount rate $r = 0.15$. Over a 15-year period the present value of consumption that does not occur because a birth has been averted was $280. However, Enke estimated that the total production surplus (undiscounted) for an average productive lifetime (age 15 to age 55) in a country with such a low per-capita income at $840. At the date of birth, with $r = 0.15$, the individual's earning stream has a present value of only $17. Thus the net benefit of preventing a birth is $263 or 2.6 times output per head.[7]

An extended version of the human investment approach was developed by George Zaidan of the World Bank.[8] Besides the present value of the unborn child's consumption, this takes into account government savings on educational expenses for that child, plus the fact that workers in the existing population would produce more per dollar paid to them because, with fewer people being born, more public funds will have been available to invest in the health and education of each of them prior to their joining the labor force. (See figure 7–1.)

One example of a cost-benefit analysis using the foregoing approach is presented in table 7–3.

In this example, discounted benefits exceed discounted costs by a considerable margin, indicating that this program was a good investment, although funding priorities depend on the benefits and costs of other worthy

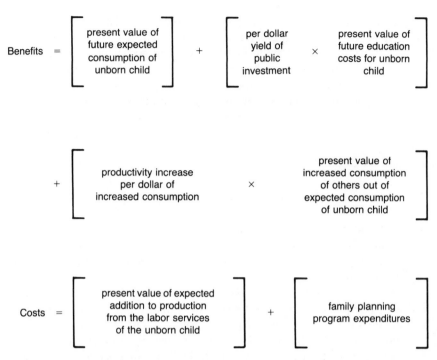

Figure 7–1. Human-investment Approach to Cost-Benefit Analysis of Family-Planning Programs

Table 7–3
Cost-Benefit of Family Planning in Egypt During the 1960s
(Egyptian £ per Prevented Birth)

	Using 10% Discount Rate	Using 15% Discount Rate
Benefits		
1. Consumption	222–351	109–206
2. Wage Productivity effect	16–21	9–14
3. Public savings effect	37	24
4. Total	275–409	142–244
Costs		
5. Productivity	79–91	24–31
6. Family planning services	4–20	4–20
7. Total	83–111	28–51
8. Differences between benefits and costs	164–326	91–216
9. Benefit/cost ratios	2.5–4.9	2.8–8.7

Source: George Zaidan, "The Costs and Benefits of Family Planning Programs," World Bank Occasional Paper no. 12 (Washington, D.C.: World Bank, 1971).

programs. (See chapter 5.) Notice that the choice of discount rate does affect the magnitude of the benefits and costs.

One serious problem with the application of cost-benefit analysis to a reduction in births is the exclusion from the calculation of psychic income that parents receive due to child rearing.[9] Moreover particularly in agrarian societies, parents may have a relatively large number of children to assure themselves of adequate support in their old age. Since these countries lack social-security systems, older persons must rely on their children for financial support.

The Macroeconomics of Population Control

The first important macroeconomic demographic model was developed by Coale and Hoover for India.[10] The model presents projections of economic and population variables from 1956 to 1986, employing three different fertility assumptions.

The primary conclusion of the Coale–Hoover study is that by 1986 income per equivalent consumer would have grown only 38 percent if high fertility prevailed throughout the period, whereas it would have grown by 95 percent if low fertility prevailed. The annual growth of income per equivalent consumer is 1.1 percent given high fertility and 2.3 percent with low fertility.

Coale and Hoover classified all expenditures into two types: developmental and nondevelopmental, or welfare expenditures. According to these authors, the welfare category of expenditures provides a lower contribution to total output. This is because the effectiveness of this category of expenditure is spread over the entire population and, because of a high dependency ratio, has little direct effect on the productivity of the labor force.

Higher fertility implies a considerable increase in welfare expenditures. In the Indian case an additional 20 to 25 billion rupees would be spent for education by 1986 (that is, over the period 1956–1986) under the high-fertility assumption as compared to the low-fertility assumption. In the Coale–Hoover model, expenditures that are used to improve the quality of labor have immediate economic impact, whereas expenditures that act upon the nonproductive population require 15 years before they have an effect on development.

A major point of the Coale–Hoover analysis is the diversion of funds to nondevelopmental outlays when fertility is high. Given the increased consumption under low fertility one would expect a positive effect on worker productivity. Coale and Hoover ignore this interaction in their analysis but this would only strengthen their conclusions. Even though the high-fertility projection involves a greater proportion of investment allocated to social welfare, the per-capita welfare expenditure is still less than with the low-fertility projection. Thus the adequacy of schools, hospitals, and housing per person is higher given expected low fertility.

In this model the main obstacle to growth is the lack of savings to finance capital formation or investment. Assuming an incremental output ratio of 3:1, it is possible to compare the required rate of investment necessary to maintain a constant per-capita income given varying hypothetical rates of population growth. If country A has a population growth rate of 1 percent, while country B has a population growth rate of 3 percent, the required rate of investment is 3 percent in A while it is 9 percent in B. The conclusion is that the required rate of saving is less likely to be realized with higher rates of population growth.

One of the important reasons why reduced population growth is expected to result in a higher rate of economic development is that a higher fraction of personal income will be saved and invested than if population growth rates remain unchanged. Increases in the rate of savings and investment tend to expand aggregate output. Since the dependents in a population ultimately must be supported by the workers, a decline in the dependency ratio is likely to cause an increase in income remaining after necessities (mainly food) have been purchased. As a result the rate of savings is expected to increase. If this happens, then the saving ratio will be negatively correlated with the rate of population growth, provided that more rapid population growth results in an increase in the dependency ratio.

It should be pointed out that the Coale–Hoover results are based on a simulation model and do not represent actual empirical findings. In recent years a number of population economists have argued that rapid population growth *enhances* economic development. Before turning to the empirical evidence, let us consider this viewpoint.

According to this approach, the Coale–Hoover analysis is clearly inadequate because it assumes that physical capital is the only factor causing an increase in per-capita output and that the input of labor is proportional to numbers in the labor force. Since physical investment is a small fraction of total output, major changes in the former mean minor changes in a large component of output like consumption. In addition, in developing countries, there is a considerable degree of nonmonetary savings, a factor frequently ignored in macroeconomic models of population and development. Moreover since the 1960s, the work of Denison,[11] Becker,[12] and Schultz[13] has emphasized the growth of knowledge and investment in human capital as being important components of economic growth. This research was stimulated by the finding that in recent years increases in physical capital and the size of the labor force account for only a small portion of the rise in GNP.

An incorrect assumption is frequently made that, as the labor force expands, an investment of new capital per person will be needed that is equal to the average capital stock per person of the present labor force. In other words the marginal capital output ratio is assumed to be equal to the average. This is unlikely to be the case, however. Many investments are indivisibile, particularly expenditures on social overhead capital such as the transportation facilities, water supply, and public buildings. These have to be provided on much the same scale for a small as for a large population. This is also true of many important industrial investments. In chemical engineering, for example, the capital cost of a plant is expressed as a power function of its intended output, the exponent of the function being as low as 0.6. This means that if one can design the plant for an increased output of, for example, 50 percent, capital requirements per unit of output will be 15 percent lower than they would have been on the smaller plant.[14]

Population growth or, to be more precise, growth of the nonfarm labor force, makes possible increased returns to scale on capital investment. Moreover, according to Clark, population growth "absolves" many countries from the harmful effects of erroneous investment decisions, whether the expenditures are private or governmental. An investment expenditure that is too large, at a given level of economic activity, can ultimately be productively used if the economy is expanding. With a stationary or declining population, however, the effect of an inappropriate investment may be a permanent economic loss.

The principal form in which economies of scale are obtained is not, as was previously believed by some, from the building of large-size facilities; it may depend more on the increased subdivision and specialization of industrial processes, which can often be achieved with relatively small plants.

Information on population growth and growth in real income per person is presented in table 7–4. Rates of population growth up to 3 percent per year seem to be increasingly positive from the point of view of improving the rate of growth of real per-capita income. Once the rate of population growth exceeds 3 percent, though, the result is a decline in real income growth.

Thirlwall analyzed available measures of population growth, productivity per person, capital stock, rates of capital investment, and also total factor productivity (the rate of growth of product per unit of inputs of both labor and capital combined in a weighted average). Thirlwall's principal finding was that there was no statistical relationship between the rate of population growth and rate of growth of capital stock or investment. This was true for both developed and developing countries. There was no support for the view that population growth and the rate of capital accumulation are inversely related in less developed countries, implying that population growth does not impede the accumulation of capital as is frequently hypothesized.

Table 7–4

Rates of Growth of Real Income, 1961–1963, to 1971–1973, Selected Countries by Rates of Population Growth

Annual Rate of Population Growth							
2.0 or Less		2.1–2.5		2.6–3.0		3.1 or More	
Angola	3.1	Egypt	1.7	Morocco	1.3	Algeria	1.8
Mozambique	3.9	Tunis	3.6	Ghana	0.4	Rhodesia	2.7
Sierra Leone	2.7	Ethiopia	2.2	Kenya	3.5	Zaire	1.6
Haiti	−0.4	Ivory Coast	5.1	Tanzania	2.6	Zambia	0.1
Jamaica	4.7	Malawi	3.4	Uganda	1.7	Costa Rica	3.2
Netherlands Antilles	−0.6	Chile	1.9	Dominican Republic	3.2	El Salvador	1.5
Argentina	3.2	Burma	0.3	Guatemala	2.8	Honduras	1.6
Uruguay	0.1	India	1.1	Nicaragua	3.1	Mexico	3.5
Mean	2.05	Sir Lanka	1.3	Panama	4.6	Columbia	2.2
		South Korea	7.5	Bolivia	2.9	Ecuador	2.3
		Mean	2.81	Brazil	3.8	Paraguay	1.5
				Malaysia	3.8	Peru	1.9
				Philippines	2.3	Syria	2.3
				Taiwan	6.9	Thailand	4.2
				Mean	3.05	Mean	2.20

Source: Colin Clark, "Population Growth and Productivity," *Research in Population Economics* 1 (1978): 143–154.

Moreover population growth in the less developed countries (LDCs) was shown to be positively associated with total factor productivity.[15]

Simon has found that higher population *density* implies faster economic growth in LDCs. According to him, this result is economically as well as statistically significant.[16] The results are drawn from a cross-section of LDCs for which data were available for 1960–1970 and 1950–1970. Simon's results agree with Strycker's recent finding for agricultural productivity in Francophone countries.[17]

In addition, total population size did not appear to affect the rate of economic growth. This apparently contradicts Chenery's (1960) findings.[18] However, it is possible that Chenery's results were due to the effects of population density rather than to total population size.

The main implication of the positive effect of population density on economic growth is that in the long run a fairly rapid rise in population would have a positive effect on per-capita income.[19] These recent studies confirm the earlier work of Easterlin[20] and Kuznets[21] in failing to show any empirical evidence that rapid population growth inhibits economic development.

None of the foregoing discussion implies that per-capita income growth *in a particular* country would have been the same if population growth rates had been markedly higher or lower However, the effect of population growth, whether positive or negative, is not so great relative to other growth determinants as to stand out in a simple comparison.

Savings and the Burden of Dependency

One of the more controversial questions in the literature is the relation-ship between the savings rate and burden of dependency. Since slower population growth reduces the burden of dependency, if higher savings were associated with a reduced burden of dependency (slower popula-tion growth) the ultimate result could be an increase in per-capita income.

An important and frequently cited study by Leff examined the associa-tion between aggregate and per-capita savings rates in relation to the burden of dependency. His sample included forty-seven developing coun-tries, twenty developed Western nations, and seven East European coun-tries. He concluded that the dependency ratios "have a statistically distinct and quantitatively important influence on aggregate savings ratios in all the countries and also within the two groups of developed and developing countries considered separately."[22] This conclusion has been strongly at-tacked by Bilsborrow, who criticized Leff's statistical methodology, as well as the choice of countries included in the aggregate sample, which, accord-ing to the former, strongly bias the results.[23] Leff's findings have been corroborated by several other investigators, however. A study by S.K. Singh, using data for seventy countries with 5-year averages to eliminate the effects of transitory phenomena, found that an increase in the dependency rate had a statistically significant effect in lowering savings rates.[24] More-over Lionel and David Demery, using data for the United Kingdom for the period 1950–1973 and applying a sophisticated economic model, found that increasing fertility led to higher aggregate consumption rates. Moreover since the aggregate consumption ratio is typically four or five times larger than the aggregate savings ratio, the impact of the dependency burden on the savings ratio was greater by the same factor.[25] Finally Kanhaya Gupta has developed a simultaneous-equation model that he estimated with data for forty developing countries. The model includes such variables as birth-rates, female labor-force participation rates, infant-mortality rates, popula-tion density, literacy, and the percentage of the labor force in agriculture. Not only did his results show the dependency rate to be a statistically significant determinant of savings rates, but Gupta concluded that Leff's single-equation model had "underestimated the depressing effect of de-pendency rate on the saving rate."[26]

The Theory of Demographic Transition

The theory of demographic transition was developed to explain the move-ment of birthrates and death rates in Western industrialized countries during the various stages of their economic development. It still presents an important framework for understanding contemporary demographic trends. (See figure 7–2.)

According to the theory of demographic transition in a preindustrial period, both fertility and mortality were at high levels. The economy was primarily agrarian, and the demographic fluctuations were primarily linked to the supply of food and the incidence of particular diseases.[27] The bulk of the population during this period achieved a standard of living that was only slightly above the subsistence level. While the population grew very slowly, severe epidemics such as that associated with the plague of 1348 (the Black Death) did result in population decline.

Stage II, which is the stage most closely associated with the theory, is the phase of demographic transition. During this phase mortality undergoes a considerable decline while fertility remains at a high level. Moreover in at

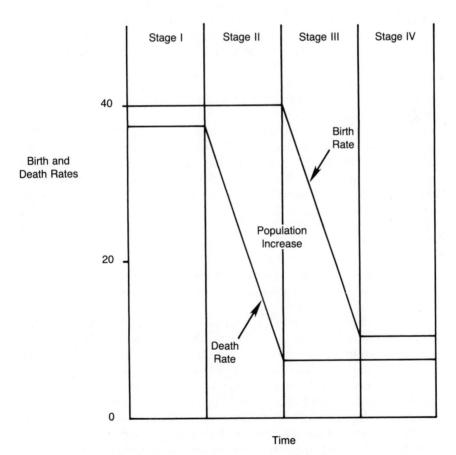

Figure 7–2. The Demographic Transition

least a few cases (Great Britain for one), fertility increases during this period.

Fertility decline commences during stage III, but only after a considerable lag with respect to the beginning of mortality decline. By the end of the third stage, most of the gap that existed between fertility and mortality levels at the beginning of this phase is eliminated.

Mortality declines initially because of the greater regularity in food supplies partly due to better transportation facilities, as well as higher production levels. The establishment of civil order and improvements in sanitation also contribute to the decline in mortality. The lag in the beginning of fertility decline results from the slowness with which contraceptive beliefs adapt to the changing environment in a developing society. Eventually however, fertility does decline in response to the occurrence of industrialization, urbanization, and the more equitable distribution of educational opportunities.

Stage II included the period of the Industrial Revolution in Western Europe. In England fertility rose initially, perhaps because children could be used as industrial wage workers to supplement the family income; and parents no longer felt as pressured to provide land for all of their children.

The most important point about the second stage of the demographic transition is that this is the phase of maximum population growth. This occurs because of the major difference between the crude birthrate and the crude death rate.

The amount of time required by a nation to complete stage II has undergone a substantial decrease. The magnitude of the decline for the countries involved seems to be associated with the date at which the demographic transition began. Thus the United States took only half as long as Western Europe to complete the demographic transition, which began considerably later as well. And Japan, whose demographic transition was completed in half the time required by the United States, began its transition even later than the United States.[28] Thus there is some evidence that for *presently developed countries* the decline in birthrates is more closely associated with the level or rate of change of per-capita income than it is with a particular time lag between the onset of the decline in death rates and the subsequent fall in birthrates.

West European countries had attained a relatively high standard of living (per-capita income) prior to the commencement of declines in birthrates. Many demographers, knowing that per-capita income levels in developing countries would not reach the level attained in Western Europe at the beginning of fertility decline for several decades, assumed that birthrates would remain at a high and constant level for many years in poor countries.

However, birthrates have declined in a number of developing countries (table 7–5). In many of these nations little economic growth has occurred. The theory of demographic transition assumed that birthrate declines were

Table 7–5
Developing Countries in Which Fertility Has Declined Appreciably,
Selected Years

Country	Crude Birthrates				Percentage Changes	
	1960	*1965*	*1970*	*1974*	*1965–1974*	*1960–1974*
Africa						
Egypt	43.6	42.1	39.4	34.8	17.3	20.1
Mauritius	40.0	35.9	28.7	25.1	30.1	37.2
Tunisia	46.6	44.7	41.4	36.0	19.4	22.8
Latin America						
Barbados	30.7	26.8	22.8	20.8	22.5	32.2
Chile	36.6	32.8	28.9	23.2	29.3	36.5
Colombia	45.3	44.2	42.1	33.0	24.4	27.2
Costa Rica	46.6	41.1	35.4	28.0	31.8	39.9
Cuba	32.4	33.1	30.2	25.3	23.5	22.0
Dominican Republic	48.5	47.2	46.4	37.5	20.6	22.7
El Salvador	48.4	46.1	43.2	40.3	12.6	16.7
Jamaica	39.4	38.5	35.3	30.6	20.5	22.3
Mexico	45.2	43.7	42.4	40.0	8.5	11.4
Panama	41.2	39.8	37.3	31.0	22.1	24.8
Trinidad and Tobago	37.7	32.5	26.6	24.0	26.2	36.2
Venezuela	45.4	42.1	37.8	36.0	14.5	20.8
Asia and the Pacific						
China	30.8	34.0	27.4	26.0	23.5	15.6
Fiji	42.0	35.7	28.5	28.0	21.6	34.1
Hong Kong	34.7	28.3	21.4	18.3	35.4	47.2
India	44.0	42.6	40.6	36.0	15.5	18.2
Indonesia	46.9	45.9	43.9	40.0	12.8	14.7
Korea	40.6	35.1	30.1	24.0	31.6	40.8
Malaysia	45.0	42.2	33.9	31.4	25.6	30.2
Philippines	44.5	44.2	44.0	37.5	15.2	15.8
Singapore	37.8	29.4	23.0	17.6	40.2	53.4
Sri Lanka	35.6	33.1	30.0	27.2	17.8	23.7
Taiwan	39.4	33.0	26.8	23.0	30.4	41.6
Thailand	46.1	44.3	43.6	34.0	23.0	26.2
Turkey	42.8	40.6	39.7	34.0	16.2	20.7
Vietnam	41.5	41.5	41.4	32.0	22.9	22.9

Adapted from Parker Mauldin and Bernard Berelson, "Cross-Cultural Review of the Effectiveness of Family Planning Programs," in *International Population Conference*, vol. 2 (Mexico City: International Union for the Scientific Study of Population, 1977), pp. 166 and 172–176.

to a considerable degree dependent on economic development. Clearly other factors are operating to reduce birthrates in developing countries. One such factor is child survival.

The Child-Survival Hypothesis

The decline in mortality of children under the age of 5 has recently been advanced as a major cause of decrease in fertility rates.[29] The most commonly stated argument is that children are an economic asset to parents—a means for assuring them support in their old age, as well as assisting in the operation of farms and other enterprises. Death of offspring contributes both directly and indirectly to fertility. If parents lose a child, they may replace that child through another birth. Moreover the risk that children may die is responsible for a form of hedging on the part of parents. In communities where infant and child mortality rates are high, parents may increase the number of births they desire as a form of insurance against the eventuality of having too few surviving children. As parents become more confident of the survival of their existing offspring, their need for additional children to ensure the minimum *declines*. Another mechanism underlying the observed mortality-fertility relationship is of biological origin. When an infant or young child dies, the mother ceases to lactate, and the probability that she will conceive increases. It is not yet clear which of the two mechanisms is more important. In any case government programs that promote reductions in mortality also tend to reduce fertility.

The child-survival hypothesis implies that declines in birthrates will lead to a fall in death rates. As a corollary of the child-survival hypothesis, one might expect that a rapid decline in death rates might shorten the interval before the birthrate commences to decline.

Taylor, Newman, and Kelly reported the distribution of the mean rate of fall in infant mortality and crude birthrates by the interval between the beginning of the fall in infant mortality (or 1945 to 1949, whichever is later) and the commencement of fertility decline for 53 countries. Of these, in only one (the Dominican Republic) was the post–World War II decline in infant mortality interrupted by a temporary rise after the beginning of fertility decline. Among the other fifty-two countries, the shorter the interval between the decline in infant mortality and the start of fertility decline, the greater has been the mean postwar rate of fall in infant mortality. For the fifty-three countries as a whole, the median interval to the beginning of fertility decline, following 1945–1949, or the subsequent start of mortality decline, is only 11.4 years.[30]

Birthrates and Economic Activity

Since children are a source of satisfaction, one might expect high-income parents to want more of them. Yet the opposite is true for several reasons. The first is that the opportunity cost of time (the time price)—earning money, developing and using skills, making use of leisure time—become more attractive as income increases. This is especially true for women, who are primarily responsible for rearing children. As opportunities for education and employment improve for women and their horizons expand, they frequently desire smaller families. As income rise, parents apparently prefer healthier and better educated, but fewer, children. They are more likely to want more education for their children when they believe that future job opportunities will be determined less by social status or family background than by education and associated skills. Since this change in attitude tends to be a consequence of economic development of nations, it is a factor explaining declining fertility over time. Finally the children of the poor work at home or outside the home at an early age. However, children from high-income families are not needed to supplement the family income. Thus Rosenzweig and Evenson, using data from India, found a significant positive relationship between the wage rates of children and birthrates, and significant negative correlations between child wages and sex-specific school enrollment rates.[31]

Rosenzweig used data from 1968 National Demographic Household Survey of the Philippines in order to indentify some of the costs and benefits of child rearing in a developing country. The econometric results suggest that in areas where child wage rates and earnings are high, parents appear to bear more children and to keep them in school for a shorter period of time than in places where child wage rates and earnings are low. Moreover children in farm households receive less schooling and engage more extensively in economic employment than urban children. The results also appear to confirm earlier findings that the schooling of the mother and the infant mortality rate of the community are important correlates of family size but they also suggest that the former variable is significantly related to child schooling attainment and employment.[32]

A study by Kasarda (cited by Rosenzweig) suggests, based on international cross-section data, that in countries with lesser utilization of child labor, birthrates are significantly lower than elsewhere. Econometric analyses of data from Puerto Rico, Egypt, Chile, Thailand, and the Philippines also contain evidence of a positive relationship between children's employment and family size.[33] While all these studies thus suggest that the economic benefits of children are clearly related to fertility, their theoretical framework is not well specified and none of the investigators provide information on the responsiveness of fertility to changes in the value of children's potential economic contributions. Nonetheless the information is crucial for policy purposes, since the value of children's services, to the extent that it is determined in the market, can be directly affected by governmental fiscal policy (taxes) or legislation regulating child labor.

Birthrates and the Distribution of Income

Birthrate declines and family-planning programs have been more successful in countries where increases in the output of goods and services have been distributed in such a way as to improve the quality of life for a substantial majority of the population rather than just for a small minority. As pointed out by Rich, the average income levels of the poorest 60 percent of the population correlate much more closely with fertility levels than do average incomes of the entire population. In a comparison of forty LDCs, an increase of $10 in the annual per-capita income of the lower 60 percent was associated with a decline of 0.7 per 1,000 in the crude birthrate, whereas a $10 increase in average income was associated with a decline of only 0.3 per 1,000.[34] These data provide further support for the hypothesis that the factor most crucial to fertility is increased distribution of income (and services) to the large low-income portion of the population.

The world fertility rate is affected by the international distribution of income in the same way that national fertility rates are affected by income distributions within countries. The same reasoning and kinds of evidence used in interpreting national fertility rates are applicable to the world fertility rate and lead to a similar conclusion. A more equal distribution of income among countries would be conducive to a lower global birthrate and a lower rate of world population growth.

This conclusion is directly related to the present world demographic situation. Thus future changes in fertility rates in the rich countries will have little influence on the global birthrate or global population growth. These depend much more heavily on future changes in birthrates in developing countries. Consequently the impact of economic growth on fertility and the rate of economic growth in the rich countries are largely irrelevant to the rate of world population change. Whatever the income fertility link is in the rich countries, it is relatively unimportant from the global perspective. What is important is the fertility decline in the poor countries and, if economic growth is conducive to that decline, then from the standpoint of world population growth only economic development in the poor countries is of importance.

From 1960 to 1978, the gap between rich and poor countries in terms of per-capita income widened. The average rate of growth in per-capita GNP was 1.6 percent from 1960 to 1978 in thirty-eight low-income countries compared to a gain of 3.7 percent in seventy middle-income and industrialized countries. In 1978 the average income in eighteen countries the World Bank classified as industrialized was $8,070 compared to $200 in the low-income countries.[35]

The greatest effect on reproduction rates is caused by increases in the per-capita income of the less developed countries. Using regression analysis, Repetto estimated the effect of income increases on the gross reproduction rate at various per-capita income levels. (See table 7–6.)

Moreover the international distribution of income and the internal distribution of income are more closely related to fertility than are the infant

Table 7-6
Estimated Marginal Effect of an Increase
of $100 in Mean per-Capita Income on the
Gross Reproduction Rate, for Countries
at Various Levels of Average per-Capita
Income

Average Per-Capita Income Level ($)	Effect on the Gross Reproduction Rate of a Rise of $100 in Average Per-Capita Income
100	−.22
200	−.20
500	−.17
1,000	−.12
1,500	−.06
2,000	−.01
3,000	+.10

Source: Robert Repetto, *Economic Equality and Fertility in Developing Countries* (Baltimore, Md.: Johns Hopkins Press, for Resources for the Future, 1979), p. 162.

mortality rate or the female literacy rate. This is important because these latter two variables are by far the more frequently considered in terms of the design of population policies. The evidence presented here supports the contention that population policies that concern themselves with the pattern of income growth and its distribution, both within and among countries, would have a greater impact than those that do not.[36]

Fertility and Economic Equality—Korea, A Case Study

Within the span of a decade, from about 1944 to 1954, Korea experienced a series of disruptive events. It emerged as a society in which economic as well as social distinctions had been reduced to a greater extent than in any noncommunist country. In fact the distribution of income at the end of this period was probably more equal than in any developing country in the world. Moreover the pattern of growth in the postwar period, based on intensive use of human resources and equal opportunity in education, has resulted in the maintenance of a great deal of that equality.

This high degree of equality was not achieved through a particularly strong commitment to social welfare but through the disruption and devastation of war. A land-reform program was implemented, however, mostly by private land sales or by the U.S. military government. Since 1953 there has been no significant redistribution.[37]

Korea provides a distinctive model among less developed countries that have undergone a substantial fertility decline. Economic policy has emphasized very rapid growth that relies heavily on imported capital and technology, the relative neglect (until recently) of agriculture in favor of nontraditional manufacturing industries producing goods for export, and a minimum of welfare programs of any kind. Economic equality has been maintained primarily by the growth of labor demand, which has expanded employment opportunities and raised real wages. Moreover the political orientation of the Korean government has not adopted policies that have favored reducing the degree of inequality in the distribution of income.

The fertility decline in Korea between 1960 and 1974 has been one of the fastest recorded in any nation in history. This suggests that what may be essential is improvement in the living standards and opportunities of the poor majority, and the absence of wide socioeconomic disparities, rather than a particular set of government policies.

The primary reason that the fertility decline Korea was so fast was that it was so pervasive. Birthrates started to decline at about the same time in all regions, classes, and categories of households. Within 6 years of the onset of the transition, fertility differentials between groups had begun to narrow, and within a decade there was substantial convergence. Shifts in the female population—from rural to urban, uneducated to educated, or economically inactive to employed—were important but by no means the predominant influences on fertility. Among the uneducated, the rural, and those within the traditional sector, birthrates also fell. Such broad participation in demographic change is characteristic of societies without marked cultural and socioeconomic differentiation.[38]

Equally broad-based were the mechanisms of fertility decline. The spread of contraception was only one means of fertility control, and, from 1960 to 1965, a relatively unimportant one. The importance of abortion and delayed marriage were more significant. It is impossible to disentangle the effects of a rising age of marriage, the growing incidence of abortion, and a more widespread use of contraceptives (obtained from private sources and from the national family-planning program), because the impact of all of these are mutually interdependent. The evidence implies that all were important. Even in rural areas the decline cannot be attributed mainly to the success of the government's family-planning program.

Despite the absence of fully satisfactory data on which to base a conclusion, the consensus is that the process of economic growth in Korea during the years of rapid expansion, 1963–1975, preserved much of the initial equality in the distribution of economic welfare. In addition, it appears that the distribution of earnings among workers in the urban sector has become, if anything, less concentrated. Earnings differentials between skilled and unskilled occupations have narrowed,[39] and the income and consumption level of wage earners have increased relative to those of salary earners.

These changes are attributable in part to the rapid growth and diffusion of education in the labor force.

In the rural sector reasonably complete data indicate an unequal and unchanging distribution of income. The share of the lowest 40 percent of farm households in total farm income has gone from 20 percent in 1963 to 19 percent in 1974. The fact that this relatively high share of income goes to persons in the lower strata does not even fully reflect the actual degree of equality, since farm households on large holdings tend to have more members.

Summary

Although birthrates have begun to fall in developing countries, population growth rates, both currently and in the near future, are expected to remain high, putting increased pressure on limited economic resources. Total world population is expected to reach 6 billion by the year 2000.

While the economic-demographic model developed by Coale and Hoover implies that population growth impedes the growth of per-capita income, Clark and Simon both disagree. The each argue that rapid population growth stimulates economic development partly because of the positive effect of economies of scale. The empirical evidence suggests that rapid population growth has a minor effect on the increase in per-capita income.

The theory of demographic transition was developed as a framework for explaining the change in birthrates and death rates in Western Europe and the United States in response to economic growth. However, birthrates in developing countries have begun to decline even when little economic improvement was occurring. This latter demographic experience has been explained with the child-survival hypothesis, which postulates that a decline in the infant-mortality rate will result in a decline in birthrates as parents become aware that fewer births are needed to assure a certain family size.

There is evidence that birthrates fall more rapidly in countries with a fairly equitable distribution of income and access to social services. Korea is presented as a case study of this relationship. The decline in birthrates in South Korea is among the fastest ever recorded.

Notes

1. The World Bank, *World Development Report, 1980* (New York, Oxford University Press, 1980), p. 64.

2. Tomas Frejka, *The Future of Population Growth* (New York: John Wiley, 1974), p. 32.

3. Ibid., p. 176.

4. Robert Repetto, *Economic Equality and Fertility in Developing Countries* (Baltimore, Md.: Johns Hopkins Press, for Resources for the Future, 1979), p. 156.

5. Ronald Freedman, "Comment" in National Bureau of Economic Research, *Demographic and Economic Change in Developed Countries* (Princeton, N.J.: Princeton University Press, 1960), p. 74; and Norman Ryder, "Recent Trends and Growth Differences in Fertility," in Charles Westoff (Ed.), *Toward the End of Growth* (Englewood Cliffs, N.J.: Prentice-Hall, 1973), p. 65.

6. Leon Tabah, "Rapport sur les Relations Entre la Fecundité et la Condition Sociale et Economique de la Famille in Europe," in Council of Europe, *Second European Population Conference* (Strasbourg: Council of Europe, 1971), p. 140.

7. Stephen Enke, "The Economic Aspects of Slowing Population Growth," *The Economic Journal* 76, no. 301 (March 1966): 44–56.

8. Nancy Yinger, Richard Osborn, David Salkever, and Ismail Sirageldin, "Third World Family Planning Programs: Measuring the Costs," *Population Bulletin* 38, no. 1 (1983): 9.

9. This point is made in R. Blandy "The Welfare Analysis of Fertility Reduction," *The Economic Journal* 84, no. 333, (March 1974): 109–129.

10. A.J. Coale and E.M. Hoover, *Population Growth and Economic Development in Low-Income Countries* (Princeton, N.J.: Princeton University Press, 1958).

11. Edward Denison, *The Sources of Economic Growth in the United States and the Alternatives Before U.S.* Supplementary Paper no. 13 (New York: Committee on Economic Development, 1962).

12. Gary Becker, *Human Capital* (New York: National Bureau of Economic Research, 1964).

13. Theodore Schultz, "Capital Formation by Education," *Journal of Political Economy* 68, no. 6 (December 1960): 571–583.

14. Colin Clark, "Population Growth and Productivity," *Research in Population Economics* I (1978): 145.

15. Thirwall's work is cited in Ibid., p. 147.

16. Julian Simon, "The Relationship between Population Growth and Economic Growth in LDCs," *Research in Population Economics* 2 (1980): 215–234.

17. J. Dirick Stryker, "Optimum Population in Rural Areas: Empirical Evidence from the Franc Zone," *Quarterly Journal of Economics*, 91, no. 2 (May 1977): 177–193.

18. Hollis B. Chenery, "Patterns of Industrial Growth," *American Economic Review* 50, no. 4 (September 1960): 624–654.

19. Simon, "Population Growth and Economic Growth in LDCs," pp. 226–227.

20. Richard Easterlin, "Effects of Population Growth on the Economic Development of Developing Countries," *Annals of the American Academy of Political and Social Science* 369, (January 1967): 6.

21. Simon Kuznets, "Quantitative Aspects of the Economic Growth of Nations," Part I, "Levels and Variability of Rates of Growth," *Economic Development and Cultural Change* 5, no. 1 (October 1956): 30.

22. Nathanial H. Leff, "Dependency Rates and Savings Rates," *American Economic Review* 59, no. 5 (1969): 893.

23. Richard Bilsborrow, "Dependency Rates and Aggregate Savings Rates Revisited: Corrections, Further Analysis, and Recommendations for the Future," *Research in Population Economics* 2 (1980): 183–204.

24. S.K. Singh, *Development Economics: Some Findings* (Lexington, Mass.: Lexington Books, D.C. Heath, 1975), pp. 133 and 149.

25. Lionel Demery and David Demery, "Demographic Change and Aggregate Consumption, U.K.: 1950–1973," in Hamish Richards (Ed.), *Population, Factor Movements and Economic Development: Studies Presented to Brinley Thomas* (Cardiff: University of Wales Press, 1976), pp. 154–179.

26. Kanhaya Gupta, "Foreign Capital Inflows, Dependency Burden, and Savings Rates in Developing Countries: A Simultaneous Equations Model," *Kyklos* 282, no. 2 (May 1975): 358–374.

27. Yves Bizien, *Population and Economic Development* (New York: Praeger Press, 1979), p. 13.

28. Ibid., p. 15.

29. See for example, Irma Adelman, "An Econometric Analysis of Population Growth," *American Economic Review* 53, no. 3 (1963): 314–339; and A. Harman, *Fertility and Economic Behavior of Families in the Philippines* RM-6385-AID (Santa Monica, Calif.: Rand, September 1970).

30. Carl Taylor, Jeanne Newman, and Narindar Kelly, "Health Aspects of Population Increase," Working Paper no. 8 for the World Population Conference, Processed, 1974, p. 15.

31. M.R. Rosenzweig and R. Evenson, "Fertility, Schooling, and the Economic Contribution of Children in Rural India: An Econometric Analysis," *Econometrica* 45, no. 5 (1977): 1065–1080.

32. Mark Rosenzweig, "The Value of Children's Time, Family Size and Nonhousehold Child Activities in a Developing Country: Evidence from Household Data," *Research in Population Economics* 1 (1979): 331.

33. Ibid., pp. 331–347.

34. Wiliam Rich, *Smaller Families through Social Economic Progress*, Monograph no. 7 (Washington, D.C.: Overseas Development Council, 1973), pp. 15–16.

35. The World Bank, *World Development Report, 1980*, pp. 110–111.

36. Repetto, *Economic Equality and Fertility in Developing Countries*, p. 162.

37. Ibid., p. 69.

38. Ibid., p. 70.

39. International Bank for Reconstruction and Development, Development Policy Staff, *Prospects for Developing Countries, 1978–1985* (Washington, D.C.: International Bank for Reconstruction and Development, 1977), p. 32.

8 Health Insurance

Health insurance is a financial mechanism for spreading the cost of medical care over as large a portion of the group at risk as possible. It is one method for removing all, or part, of the economic barrier to health and medical-care services. The fundamental justification for health insurance is the uneven and unpredictable incidence of illness that leads to wide fluctuations in medical-care expenditures at a point in time. One purpose of health insurance is to equalize the distribution of the burden of medical-care costs among individuals and families. Because health insurance entails a transfer of purchasing power from the well to the sick, it increases the total demand for services. It also assures that the producer will be paid for services rendered.

Insurance is a means for reducing the uncertainty of economic loss that is associated with a random event. The possibility of loss is transferred from the individual policyholder to an insurance company. The latter reimburses the policyholder for all or part of the losses resulting from a particular occurrence. Insurance companies pool the risks of many people so that they can predict fairly accurately the level of claims. Moreover commercial insurance companies make a profit by charging a premium in excess of the expected claims filed by policyholders.[1]

One should note the distinction between prepayment and insurance. Regular expected services, such as an annual physical exam, may be prepaid but not insured. Occasional unexpected services may be both prepaid and insured. With respect to regularly expected services, the cost to the patient, if he attempted to insure for these expenses, would be higher than if he paid for them at the time services were rendered. This is because, with utilization being certain, the insurance company would have to charge a premium that would be the sum of the reimbursable cost for services rendered plus a loading charge.

Basic Principles of Health Insurance

To operate successfully, insurance policies must be structured to minimize moral hazard, keep administrative costs as low as possible, and to establish

167

premiums that reflect the risk to the insured.[2] *Moral hazard* refers to actions of the insured person in seeking to gain reimbursement under the insurance contract that increases the likelihood of the insurer incurring a loss. In the most severe form of moral hazard, the policyholder may directly cause the loss in order to be reimbursed by the insurance company. A subtler form of moral hazard occurs when the insured increases demand for service because its marginal cost has been reduced to zero or near zero (because the person is insured). For example, an insured person might visit a doctor for a minor illness but would treat himself if he had to pay the full cost of the visit. In addition, he might influence his physician to order many expensive specialized tests while he is hospitalized if the ancillary procedures are fully covered by insurance. One means of reducing moral hazard is to have the insured bear part of the cost of any medical expense through deductible or coinsurance features.

A deductible is a specific dollar amount of the bill that must be paid by the insured. Thus an insurance policy with a $100 deductible means the initial $100 of cost is paid by the insured. Coinsurance refers to a situation where the holder of the insurance policy pays a specific proportion of the total bill. Thus a policy with 20 percent coinsurance would mean that if the total bill were $1,000, the insured would have to pay $200.

A second principle of sound insurance practice is to keep administrative costs, which must be added to the actuarily determined fair premium, as low as possible. Incentives are needed to reduce the number of claims, since these require paperwork and staff time. The insurance policy should be structured so that small (relatively frequent) economic losses are not reimbursable. One way of reducing the number of claims is to put a deductible clause in the insurance policy so that persons with small losses do not file claims because they will not be reimbursed.

Finally, insurance policies must reflect insurance risks. Someone in poor health may be charged a higher premium than a person whose health status is higher. Since poor health status is more frequently associated with low income, this insurance principle may cause problems of equity, although the latter is a separate matter.

These basic principles are just as relevant for medical insurance as for other types, but for a number of reasons they are frequently ignored.[3] Most hospitalization insurance covers all expenses that are incurred so the insured has no financial incentive to reduce costs. The patient's out-of-pocket costs are unaffected should his physician order unnecessary laboratory tests, x-ray examinations, or other services. Moreover, since many subscribers have their entire premium paid by their employer, they are unconcerned (in the short run) about rapidly rising insurance premiums due to increasing hospital costs. Since most hospital insurance has no deductible provision, some relatively small claims cost more to process than the actual amount of the bill. Even though most types of insurance policies have deductible or coinsurance features, it is not common practice to write such policies for hospital insurance.[4] Moreover some people are covered by two or more policies, so that they actually profit financially if they are hospitalized. In addition, physicians frequently have patients hospitalized who could have been treated on an out patient basis because those patients have only hospitalization insurance.

Besides the lack of incentive for reducing hospital costs, hospital insurance does not typically have a maximum amount per claim; thus the insured can obtain care of any quality or cost, which can result in very high charges. Finally, most hospital-insurance plans are inequitable in that there is little choice regarding coverage for members within a group, and all members generally pay the same premium regardless of age or sex, both of which significantly affect the risk of hospitalization and its associated costs. These inequities may be justified as a means of reducing the premiums of the elderly and the chronically ill; but this point is unrelated to the issue of insurance and violates the third of the aforementioned guidelines regarding appropriate insurance practice. There is no good reason to merge considerations of health-insurance efficiency with questions of income redistribution, although some proponents of particular national health insurance proposals would vigorously disagree.

Some economists maintain that medical care has particular features that exclude it from the typical insurance criteria.[5] It is maintained that patients have no role in decision making regarding their demand for medical services. Instead it is physicians who use their medical judgment to determine their patients' demand for medical care. Decisions regarding hospitalization or otherwise, length of stay, and choice of hospital, are supposedly made without regard to the patient's insurance status so that moral hazard is absent.

While a number of researchers have emphasized that physicians as well as administrators significantly affect hospital utilization and costs, it is clear that many patients do have some influence on demand.[6] A patient with no insurance may resist spending 3 days in a hospital (at $200 per day) to undergo diagnostic tests that could readily be performed on an out-patient basis. With complete insurance coverage the patients may still object to spending time in the hospital but are less likely to question the recommended hospitalization, especially if they receive paid sick leave from their jobs (another form of full-pay medical-insurance coverage). The patient who has vague occasional discomfort and requests medical treatment will probably be required to undergo a battery of laboratory tests. The insured patient is likely to feel entitled to the highest quality care because of having paid the insurance premium. In this situation only the doctor's restraint and the demands of other patients for hospital services may limit the patient's expenditures.

The price of insurance to an individual is the ratio of insurance premiums to expected or average dollar benefits he or she might receive. The difference between premiums and the level of benefits represents the selling and administrative costs of the insurance provider. When insurance is provided to employees as a group rather than to each one individually, there is a substantial saving on selling and administrative costs, and lower premiums result. The premium per insured for group insurance is generally 50 to 80 percent less than the premium for identical benefits if the insurance were purchased individually.[7] The advantage of group purchasing of insurance increases with firm or group size. While there could be some disadvantages to group insurance—individuals may not be able to get precisely the kind of insurance policy they want—it is generally found that relatively few persons who lack access to group policies actually purchase individual insurance policies.

In addition to the lower cost of group insurance, the part of the insurance premium paid by the employer is in effect tax-free income. Thus the person obtains the same insurance policy whether the employer buys it or whether the employer pays the worker the equivalent dollar value which the worker then uses to purchase the same policy. However, the employee who receives the money as income must pay tax on it, whereas if the employer pays the premium, the cost of the policy is not included as income and therefore is not taxed. This is clearly a major incentive for purchasing insurance. In addition, the tax benefits are so substantial that for all but the least-paid workers, it is actually less costly on average to buy medical care via insurance than to purchase it when the need arises (self-insure). Thus the tax savings from having medical care paid for by one's employer via his paying the insurance premium rather than paying for the care out of after-tax income *exceed* the costs of administering insurance and processing claims. While this saving is positive for almost all workers, it is clearly related to the worker's income and resultant tax burden, as well as the increase in his medical expense. Since there is a tendency for both the tax rate and medical expenses to increase with income, the incentive to purchase insurance increases with income.[8]

Insurance also performs a budgeting function; it allows people to save for medical expenses on a regular basis free of taxes. One alternative is to borrow funds to pay medical expenses, but for most consumers this possibility is generally not available, at least at reasonable interest rates.

Young workers are less likely to be insured than older workers, partly because the former are more likely to be employed part time. The probability of being hospitalized while young is less than that for a middle-aged person, but insurance premiums are generally the same for both. Thus for the young, insurance is relatively much less advantageous; it is not surprising that insurance enrollment rates are lower for young as compared to middle-aged workers.

Why, especially for hospital expenses, is coverage frequently more common for short hospital stays (first-dollar coverage), but less common in terms of catastrophic expenses? First, almost everyone has some type of catastrophic coverage provided by some level of government. Because large medical and dental expenses are deductible in the federal (and some state) income taxes, there is a tax subsidy to catastrophic expenditures. For lower-income persons, catastrophic medical expenses often make people eligible for public or private charity, although if private insurance benefits are available, they must be used first.

Second, from the viewpoint of the provider, hospitalization insurance (via the Blue Cross approach) was originally developed by hospitals to assist them in collecting their bills during the depression. A much higher proportion of a hopsital's bills involve first-dollar as opposed to catastrophic coverage. Thus Blue Cross has not aggressively marketed major medical insurance.[9]

Most bills for hospital care and in-hospital physicians' services are already covered by third-party payments. One would expect that the small increase involved in moving to full coverage under national health insurance would have a modest effect on total hospital expenditures. One study estimated that in-patient expenditures under national health insurance would rise only 15 percent compared to a much larger increase for ambulatory services.[10]

One important consideration is that presently uninsured persons, even though few in number, may be the only important constraint on the increase in utilization and expenditures in hospitals. If this restraining influence is eliminated, cost increases may accelerate.

Because consumers pay only a tiny fraction of total hospital costs, they will demand (or be willing to accept) greater improvements in quality than would be the case if they were uninsured and had to pay the full cost. Given the present system of third-party reimbursement, the opportunity exists for hospitals and doctors to emphasize quality improvements. The high cost of medical care induces people to buy more insurance coverage, but the additional coverage (by raising demand) tends to push prices still higher.[11]

One may consider a system in which the individual physician or all practicing physicians in the hospital as a group bear some of the risk of higher hospital costs initially. Thus costs greater than some target figure would to some extent be charged to the physician or physicians. The target could be based on statistical determination of appropriate or average charges per unit of output, or the indemnity character of this arrangement could be made explicit, with consumers being able to choose their preferred level of indemnity. Once the excess charges are billed to the physician, he may subsequently wish to bill patients for them. This should make the patients more cost conscious and interested in the usefulness of the care provided. The important point is that the physician should not be allowed to obtain insurance reimbursement for these excess charges.

With respect to hospital care, the general problem is not too little insurance coverage; it is that there is too much of the wrong type of insurance. Most national health-insurance plans will just add the last increments of the same kind of coverage that is readily available. If this legislation goes into effect, it may have a severe effect by removing the last significant constraint on hospital costs. Restrictions on providers or planning controls would clearly be necessary once market forces were eliminated.

The incentives in terms of third-party reimbursement also prevent local efforts to control costs by limiting hospital capacity. Most of the costs of operating excess hospital capacity are paid by Medicare, Medicaid, and insurance policies whose premiums are based on rated experience of an area larger than a typical county or health service area. Why should a health-systems agency or a board of county supervisors resist local pressures and force the closing of an unneeded hopsital, or at least a reduction in its capacity, with attendant loss of jobs, when most of the funds necessary for keeping it at its present size come from sources outside their area?

Most private health insurance is provided as an employment-related fringe benefit—a system that works fairly well for a large proportion of the economically self-sufficient population with job stability (except that a limit on the number of employer health-plan offerings is a major obstacle to competition and consumer choice). However, the employment-health insurance linkage is not compatible with an effective universal system of insurance coverage because people lose their insurance when they are laid off. Employment changes usually require a new insurance policy or prepaid plan with breaks in continuity of coverage and care. Moreover it is very difficult to provide good insurance coverage for persons in low-profit, highly competitive industries or in firms with seasonal, intermittent or otherwise unstable levels of employment. Furthermore, employer-employee financing has a regressive impact. Without mandated employer-provided coverage, the low paid, who often need the most protection, get the least; however, with mandated coverage, in addition to considerable administrative problems covering workers with unstable employment, a strong disincentive would be created for employing low-productivity workers.[12]

Private Insurance Plans

Variations in purchasing power, compounded by insurers' incentives to limit their exposure to financial risk, have divided the insurance market into large employee groups and the remainder of the population. There are several reasons why large groups obtain broad coverage at relatively low rates. Favorable tax treatment of employers' contributions to insurance premiums, the reduction in risk associated with large numbers of persons in relatively good health, and the sheer volume of premium dollars have all combined to make employees of large unionized industries quite attractive to insurance companies. Competition to insure these groups has helped to minimize administrative costs and provided an incentive for insurers to relate rates exclusively to costs incurred by each group's members, that is, to utilize "experience rating" instead of "community rating," under which members of different groups are charged the same premium. Since employed people are generally healthier than others in the population, experience rating means that workers' groups pay lower premiums than they would if they absorbed some of the health costs of the unemployed and those not in the labor force. Better health status and lower administrative costs per person in large employee groups also make their insurance premiums lower than for those for small groups and individuals.[13]

The availability of insurance through employment is a function of firm size. A 1977–78 Battelle survey found that only 50 percent of firms with between two and nine employees offered group health insurance, as compared with 85 percent of firms with ten to ninety-nine employees, and 100 percent of firms employing one hundred or more workers.[14]

Although limitations exist, a rising proportion of large group policies are aligning benefits to full service costs and increasing lifetime ceilings. In 1976, 90 percent of workers in group plans in firms with twenty-five or more employees reportedly had "major medical" benefits, which pay the major part (usually) 80 percent of charges for most medical services after beneficiaries meet an initial deductible. These plans offer lifetime maximum benefits ranging from under $10,000 to $250,000 or more, with a growing number of policies providing unlimited benefits. In 1976, however, less than 10 percent of workers in group plans in firms with more than 25 employees had unlimited benefits.[15] Although most major medical plans have coinsurance features (usually 20 percent of charges after a deductible), a growing number of plans set limits on the beneficiaries' out-of-pocket payments, thereby providing significant protection against catastrophic costs. Roughly 20 percent of employees in group plans in firms with more than twenty-five employees had coverage of this kind in 1976[16]

Part-time employees, the self-employed, and the unemployed have limited access to group insurance policies. Health insurance, like other fringe benefits, may not be available to part-time employees, and unemployed workers may lose their group health benefits after they are laid off or resign. Table 8–1 indicates the percentages of each of these groups and of full-time workers with group health benefits in 1976. The unemployed have better insurance coverage than anticipated because some group health insurance plans maintain benefits during short-term layoffs.

Table 8-1

Percentages of Persons with and without Insurance Protection, 1976

	Percentage of Poulation		With No Private Health Insurance	With neither Private nor Public Health Coverage
	With Group Insurance	With Individual Insurance		
Age				
Less than 19 years	65.4	12.2	24.4	——
19–24	58.0	14.6	29.0	20.5
25–44	72.3	13.7	17.7	9.3
45–64	66.6	20.8	16.5	7.6
65 and over	18.3	38.7	38.7	1.0
Family income				
Less than $5,000	30.8	39.3	26.9	17.4
$5,000–$9,999	43.5	20.4	36.7	16.6
$10,000–$14,999	70.1	15.8	16.6	9.2
$15,000 or more	79.3	15.3	9.2	5.7
Employment status				
Full-time wage earner	82.6	13.1	9.6	6.5
Part-time wage earner	63.2	18.5	20.0	12.1
Self-employed	33.0	41.3	24.6	14.9
Unemployed	41.5	14.9	44.9	26.8
Retired	26.2	34.4	36.0	2.0
Not in labor force	55.8	16.4	29.0	11.4
Total	61.9	17.2	23.0	5.7–9.0

Source: U.S. Congress, Congressional Budget Office, *Profile of Health Care Coverage: The Haves and Have-Nots* (Washington, D.C.: U.S. Government Printing Office, 1979), tables 1 and 11, pp. 2 and 24.

Table 8-2

Enrollment in Insurance Companies' Health Policies, 1978

(Persons under Age 65)

Expenses Covered	Group Policies	Individual and Family Policies
Hospital care	84,857,000	29,155,000
Surgical services	94,109,000	15,149,000
Physicians' expense protection	90,208,000	12,450,000
Major-medical expense protection	97,187,000	6,715,000

Source: Health Insurance Institute, *Source Book of Health Insurance Data, 1979–1980* (Washington, D.C.: Health Insurance Institute, 1980), pp. 13–17.

People with limited access to group health insurance have the option of purchasing individual health-insurance policies. However, the latter generally offer fewer benefits at higher costs than the former. Table 8–2 compares the enrollment (for persons under age 65) by policy type for group and individual policies in 1978. The number of enrollees with group policies does not decline with the expanding scope of coverage. However, enrollment in individual policies declines sharply as benefits expand, indicating that most individuals purchase only limited coverage.

Not only are types of coverage more limited with individual as compared to group policies, but restrictions within types of coverage are greater for the former. Finally, as mentioned previously, premiums for insurance companies' individual policies reflect extremely high administrative costs. In 1977, insurance companies spent only 54.2 percent of premium incomes for benefits under individual plans, retaining the remainder to cover operating expenses and profits. This compares with a retention rate of 13.6 percent under group policies.[17]

Table 8–1 illustrates that group coverage varies with employment status, income, and age. More than 50 percent of the uninsured population have incomes less than $10,000, and almost 75 percent have incomes below $15,000. Moreover, group coverage is more limited among persons between 19 and 24 years old than for any other age group except the elderly. This reflects the fact that many policies terminate coverage of dependents when they reach 18 years of age, unless they are in school.

Public Insurance Plans

The inadequacies of in private insurance coverage have long been recognized and were an important factor in the passage of Medicare and Medicaid legislation in 1965. Medicare is a federal health-insurance program for people 65 or older and certain disabled people. It is operated by the Health Care Financing Administration.

Medicare has two parts—hospital insurance and medical insurance. Hospital insurance helps to pay for in-patient hospital care, in-patient care in a skilled nursing facility, and home health care. Medical insurance can help pay for medically necessary doctors' services, out-patient hospital services, and a number of other medical services and supplies that are not covered by the hospital insurance part of Medicare. Medical insurance also can pay for home health services.

Hospital insurance pays for up to 90 days of medically necessary in-patient hospital care. There is a $260 deductible. From the sixty-first to the ninetieth day of hospitalization, Medicare will pay for all covered services except for $65 a day. In addition, during your *lifetime*, you are alloted 60 reserve days to supplement hospital stays that exceed 90 days. For reserve days the hospital insurance pays for all covered services except for $130 per day for each reserve day used.

Regarding medical insurance under Medicare, there is a $75 deductible and a coinsurance rate of 20 percent. The basic medical insurance premium is $12.20 a month as of July 1, 1982.[18] Under the law the premium can be raised only if there has been a general increase in Social Security cash benefits during the previous year. Medicare provides relatively compre-hensive—though far from complete—insurance protection for almost all citizens aged 65 and over. A comparison of columns 3 and 4 for persons 65 and older in table 8–2 reveals the significant effect that Medicare has had on insurance protection for the elderly. In 1976 38.7 percent of this group had no private insurance, but only 1 percent had no insurance at all. As indicated previously, Medicare also covers medical costs for individuals who have received Social Security disability benefits for 2 years. The coverage ulti-mately protects people who are unable to work because of illness. However, the 2-year waiting period leaves the disabled exposed to potentially cata-strophic expenditures.

Medicaid was intended to protect people who are too poor to afford private insurance and in some states people who become poor because of illness (the "medically needy"). Unfortunately Medicaid's design leaves many people in both categories unprotected. (See chapter 9 for further information on this point.)

Health-Maintenance Organizations

For purposes of analysis, a health-maintenance organization (HMO) must have the following five essential features:[19]

1. The HMO assumes a contractual responsibility to provide or ensure the delivery of specific kinds of health services, including, as a minimum, physician and hospital services.
2. The HMO provides medical care for those persons enrolled in the health plan.
3. Enrollment in the health plan (HMO) is voluntary.
4. The HMO requires a fixed periodic payment to the organization that is independent of the volume of health services consumed. (There may be small charges related to utilization, but these are generally minor.)
5. The HMO bears at least part of the financial risk or gain in the provision of services.

There are basically two types of HMOs. The first is known as a prepaid group practice. The second type is termed an individual practice association. Although there are some exceptions, most group plans compensate their physicians on a salary or capitation basis, while most individual practice associations comprise physicians in private offices who bill the HMO on a fee-for-service basis.[20]

HMO Costs

HMOs are potentially useful as a means for cost control because they change the standard economic incentives in medical care and motivate providers to limit costs. The evidence is consistent with this hypothesis, particularly when the response to HMO incentives is compared with the present system of extensive third-party reimbursement for providers. In all cases the total cost of medical care (premium plus out-of-pocket costs) for HMO enrollees is lower than for comparable people with health insurance coverage.[21] The lower costs are most evident for enrollees in prepaid group practices, where total costs range from 10 to 40 percent below those incurred by participants in conventional insurance programs. Although the evidence is limited, costs for enrollees in individual practice associations are approximately the same as for enrollees in conventional plans. (See table 8–3.)

The main reason for cost differences is not lower cost per unit of service rendered but differences in utilization of services. Based on the studies indicated in table 8–3, there is strong evidence for the claim that enrollees in group practices have lower hospitalization rates than do people with conventional insurance. However, the results for individual practice association enrollees are ambivalent. Average differences in utilization by enrollees in HMOs and by persons who rely on fee-for-service medical care are substantial, with about 30 percent fewer hospital days for enrollees in prepaid group practices, and 20 percent fewer days for enrollees in individual practice associations. HMO enrollees have a somewhat shorter hospital stay than do people in conventional plans, but most of the overall utilization difference stems from lower admission rates.

If one ignores the impact of specific organizational features, there are two primary explanations for these lower admission rates: (1) that HMOs identify and treat as out-patients those persons who do not require hospitalization—the discretionary and perhaps unnecessary cases; and (2) that HMOs obtain a lower hospitalization rate than nonenrollees without any apparent discrimination according to obvious necessity.

The best available data from a wide variety of HMOs tend to support the second explanation instead of the first. HMOs do not achieve a disproportionate share of their lower admission rates by reducing surgical as opposed to medical cases. Instead admissions are lower for both types of patients. In addition, while admissions for certain discretionary procedures, such as hernia repair and hysterectomy, are lower in HMOs than in conventional insurance plans, the figures for discretionary procedures do not appear disproportionately lower than the data for all surgery. The measures of discretionary care are very rough approximations that blur the subtle distinctions in patient care, however. Thus many so-called discretionary admissions are likely essential and many nondiscretionary admissions are really optional.[22]

Table 8–3
Ratios of Utilization and Cost Measures in Health-Maintenance Organizations to Those in Fee-for-Service Independent Practices, Selected Studies

| | Hospital | | Physician | | |
Study	Admissions	Days	Visits	Surgical Procecures	Total Costs
Denson et al. 1958	.86	.91	—	.82	—
Anderson and Sheatsley 1959	.57	.47	.92	.65	.90
Densen et al. 1960	.80	.78	—	.79	—
Falk and Senturia 1960	.85	.55	.77	.48	—
	.77	.40	1.61	.52	—
Densen et al. 1962	1.01	1.00	—	—	—
Williams et al. 1964	1.04	1.05	1.32	1.05	.86
	1.11	1.00	1.13	1.61	.89
Dozier et al. 1964	.65	.81	1.06	—	.77
Shapiro et al. 1967	—	.87	.98	—	—
Chamberlain 1967	.60	.53	—	—	—
National Advisory Commission 1967	.68	.69	.94	—	.54
Perrott and Chase 1968	.50	.47	—	.42	—
Perrott 1971	.49	.49	—	.45	—
Robertson 1972	.49	.40	2.13	.33	—
Hastings et al. 1973	.80	.76	1.48	—	—
Broida 1975	1.54	1.41	2.29	—	—
Reidel et al. 1975	.57	.58	—	—	—
Wersinger et al. 1976	.64	.63	—	—	—

Source: Frederic Wolinsky, "The Performance of Health Maintenance Organizations: An Analytic Review," *Milbank Memorial Fund Quarterly* 58, no. 4 (Fall 1980): 556.

Quality of Care

Improved health status or outcome is the objective of medical care. Unfortunately changes in health status are very difficult to measure. Health-service investigators therefore rely on indirect measures of medical-care quality, such as the presence of particular resources (structural measures) and the use of correct procedures for given cases (process measures). There is little evidence that structure, process, and health-status measures correlate well with each other or with what people might accept as quality indicators.[23]

In terms of structural measures, existing data indicate that HMOs have resources of equal quality with that provided by conventional insurance plans to enrollees. HMOs tend to have higher proportions of more highly trained physicians and are more likely to use accredited hospitals.

Although HMOs have higher quality than conventional practitioners when process measures (especially laboratory costs and procedures) are used, this result appears to reflect comprehensiveness of coverage rather than organizational features. Large, prepaid group practices often deliver higher-quality services than do average fee-for-service providers, but the quality is not noticeably higher than what comparable size fee-for-service groups provide.

Outcome measures are of crucial importance in quality evaluation; the available studies focus on narrowly defined mortality-morbidity measures or on broad measures such as disability days. The initial studies of the Health Insurance Plan of Greater New York indicated lower prematurity and mortality rates for HMO enrollees.[24] However, more recent research is inconclusive. In general the available data suggest that outcomes in HMOs are similar or somewhat better than those obtained in conventional practice.

Thus although the quality issue has not been resolved, there is no evidence that HMOs achieve their utilization and cost savings by offering substantially lower-quality care than fee-for-service providers. In fact there is some evidence that HMOs provide higher-quality care.[25]

National Health Insurance—Historical Background

The first major involvement of the U.S. government with illness and the provision of medical care for other than the armed services occurred very early in the nation's history. It began with the Marine Hospital Service Act in 1798, to provide for sick or disabled merchant seaman.[26] Initially it was a compulsory contributory national sickness insurance program for a particular category of employed persons. In later years it was supported by federal expenditures.

The first major campaign for provision of health insurance by state government was undertaken from 1912 to 1920 by the American Association for Labor Legislation. This organization had recently succeeded in obtaining the enactment of workmen's compensation laws to provide protection for employees sustaining work-connected accidents and injuries. The association was attempting to obtain corresponding protection unconnected with the work place. This campaign was unsuccessful and was doomed after the American Medical Association and other early supporters retracted their previous support and blocked legislative action in the sixteen states that considered relevant proposals.[27]

In the early 1920s concern was expressed by academic experts and other concerned persons that the medical-care delivery system was becoming increasingly inadequate. Thus knowledgeable persons in medicine, public health, economics, and sociology believed it important to assess the trends in the development of the health care system and to recommend appropriate policies. The result was the formation of the Committee on the Costs of Medical Care.

During the 5 years of its existence, the committee produced a large number of monographs dealing with various economic aspects of health care. Its final report presented five major recommendations that in total constituted the first statement regarding a national health program:[28]

1. For better organization of personal health services, especially through comprehensive group practice.
2. For strengthening of the public health services.
3. For group payment of the costs, whether through nonprofit insurance, taxation, or combinations.
4. For more effective coordination of the services.
5. For improvement of professional education, with increasing emphasis on the teaching of health and the prevention of disease.

Partly as a result of the severe economic depression that was affecting the country in 1932 (when the report was released), as well as the strong opposition of organized medicine, the recommendations attracted little public support.

The Committee on Economic Security established by President Roosevelt in 1934 proposed a broad national health program to be included in the Social Security Act. However, it was believed that inclusion of such proposals would make it more difficult to pass the Social Security legislation. Thus most facets of the national health program were excluded because of political expediency.

President Roosevelt had permitted the Social Security Board to continue to propose national health program developments during the war years but did not press for enactment. When Harry Truman became president, he pressed for enactment of national health insurance in terms of a series of annual Wagner–Murray–Dingell Bills, and expressed his personal views in a succession of health messages to Congress (1945, 1947, and 1949); but he could not overcome the opposition. There was continuing legislative opposition to national health insurance (NHI).[29]

Although President Truman repeated his request in 1950, national compulsory health insurance soon disappeared as a significant legislative issue. It reemerged about 10 years later in the form of health insurance for the elderly. Beginning in the late 1960s, the movement for national health insurance again gained momentum with over thirty differing bills dealing with this issue being introduced during the 1970s.

National Health Insurance—Some General Principles

Almost all national health insurance legislation specifies a mix of direct (cost-shared) and indirect (prepaid) financing. When cost-sharing is based on the quantity of services or on the level of medical expenditure, it helps divert medical care and health-insurance benefits to high-income persons at the expense of low- or moderate-income individuals. When indirect payments or premium levels are determined by insurance risks rather than by income, they may be too high for persons with moderate means and are likely to exclude such persons from the national insurance program. If, as indicated previously, health insurance is linked to salaried employment, it tends not to include the unemployed and the self-employed. In order to minimize this inequity, some NHI proposals have specified separate insurance plans for the disadvantaged. Such programs, which require income-limits to determine eligibility, have the unfortunate effect of creating disincentives for people to earn more than the maximum amount for which one can still be eligible for benefits.

The principle of insurance implies that either all or most of the funds required to finance covered services are obtained through prepayment. The prepayment amounts can be termed *premium* or *tax*. When a premium is required by the government, it is compulsory and is in effect a tax. If a portion of the covered medical services are directly paid or partly paid by the consumers of the services, then the level of the premium or tax levy can be reduced accordingly. Thus a high level of coinsurance by the users of medical facilities can substantially reduce the level of premiums paid by all insured persons.[30]

Indirect or prepaid financing of medical services can take the form of a premium or a tax based either on insurance risk or on income. As mentioned previously, the premium levels set by private insurance organizations are experience-rated; they are based on insurance risks, and are designed to reflect differences in protection because of these risks. Premiums that are determined by risk can vary a great deal among persons with equal income; or they can be equal for persons with very different income levels. For any given level of risk, the burden of paying such a premium lessens as income rises. Alternatively, premium levels that increase with income distribute the burden equitably. However, such income-related payments require information on individual incomes. Because of its authority to collect income taxes, the government is legally entitled to such information, and no one else is entitled to it. Thus, in effect, the government is the only institution that can obtain an equitable sharing of medical-care costs.

The problem of equity in indirect financing was an issue with respect to every piece of national health insurance legislation. Some bills stipulated that premium levels should be proportional to income or earnings at least up to a specified maximum level. Thus the size of the premium was determined on a basis that applied equally to the entire population, with the federal government collecting the premiums. Other bills specified that premiums were to be paid to private insurance organizations. The bills in this group specified what proportion of the premium was directly paid by the policy-holders and what share was paid by them indirectly through their employers. The amount of the premium was based on negotiation between the policy-holders or their employers and the insurance carriers. Enrollment in the private insurance plan was generally voluntary for the employee but manda-tory for the employer. Individuals who were either self-employed or unem-ployed could have purchased individual policies but would have had to pay premium levels that were above those in group insurance policies. Thus such premium levels paid for private insurance protection reflected not only disparities in risk but also differences in employment status.[31]

To counteract the inequitable effect of fixed premiums that were high relative to earnings for low-income persons, some bills specified direct and explicit subsidies. However, means tests, or income tests, would have had to be used to determine eligibility. As mentioned earlier, these subsidies would have created so-called notch problems similar to those that have caused dissatisfaction with many antipoverty programs. Moreover though many national health insurance bills have proposed these subsidies for the poor and near poor, they also permitted an indirect subsidy through the federal income tax, vis-à-vis the premiums paid under the regular employer-employee and individual plans. Thus while the explicit subsidies for premi-ums paid by the low- and moderate-income groups were expected to decline as income increases, the implicit, or tax-related, subsidies actually increased with income. However, premiums collected as a social insurance tax are not tax exempt.

As indicated previously, the most prevalent form of private insurance is group insurance through employment. In this case the employer has the responsibility for negotiating the premium levels with the insurance organi-zation and for collecting premiums on behalf of the latter. Premiums are determined according to the degree of insurance risk, which is based on the past experience of the group. Since an employer often pays directly a high percentage of the premium, the present situation provides an incentive for both the insurer and the employer to exclude high-risk persons from the insurance plan. Moreover, if such exclusion is not feasible, there is strong incentive not to hire someone in poor health who would likely be a high risk. Most bills specified that an individual who was not an employee could have qualified for an individual policy or enrolled in a government plan. However, individual policyholders would have had to pay much higher premium levels than participants in a group plan. Depending on insurance risk and employment status, premium levels could be high relative to income for persons slightly above the poverty level.

Cost sharing can include deductibles or coinsurance or an upper limit may be placed either on the insurer's liability or on the patient's requirement for medical payments. All bills considered by Congress placed some upper limit on the patient's liability, but they differed with respect both to the method of determining the ceiling and the level of the ceiling itself. Compared to the present situation, in which the patient's liability is often unlimited and the insurer has a ceiling, any of the proposed provisions for insurance protection against catastrophic expenses would constitute a net gain.[32]

When cost sharing is based either on the level of charges or on the number of units of service utilized, it is unrelated to income. If cost sharing amounts are the same at different income levels, they comprise a decreasing portion of income as income increases. Thus their restraining effect of cost sharing gradually declines as income levels rise. Hence high-income persons are likely to exceed the level of initial deductible and to reach a fixed income limit of catastrophic protection more often than persons who, because of their low or moderate income, are deterred by the cost-sharing provisions. Therefore, if cost-sharing amounts are based on the level of charges or use, a proportionally larger share of benefits from the national health insurance program would therefore be diverted to high- or middle-income persons at the expense of those or persons with low or moderate incomes.

Those who advocate cost sharing as a policy tool desire it not only as a source of payment for medical care but also as a device for rationing demand. As such it is designed to limit the increase in demand that could be stimulated by extending appropriate insurance coverage to more persons. However, several of the bills that stipulated cost sharing also allowed or even provided incentives for private supplementary insurance that would cover the expenditures for deductibles and copayments incurred under national health insurance.

A national health insurance program, if financed solely through prepayments, would be expected to increase the overall demand for medical services and especially the demand for services that have generally not been covered by insurance.[33] Such demand increases would likely be caused both by an increase in the number of persons using services, as well as from the quantity of services used by each person. Demand pressures may be felt more strongly in the short run than in the long run because pent-up demand would largely be satisfied after a few years. However, if the short-run supply of services did not keep pace with the increase in demand, the equilibrating mechanism could result in rising costs or longer waits for appointments.

Those who favor direct patient participation in paying medical expenses hope to make consumers cost conscious and give them a strong incentive to resist the rising cost of health care services. Evidence from cross-sectional studies, based on microdata, suggests that expenditures for such services is sensitive to cost-sharing amounts and income levels. For example, Phelps and Newhouse estimated that introducing a coinsurance rate of 25 percent reduced the services consumed by professionals less than the services rendered to nonprofessionals.[34] In other words coinsurance not only limits utilization for services for consumers at all income levels but has a more restrictive impact on low- or moderate-income consumers than on those with higher incomes.

One way of dealing with this inequity is for cost-sharing amounts to be adjusted to reflect income differences over the entire income distribution and not only for the very poor and medically indigent proportion of the population. But such an adjustment would be difficult and expensive to put in practice. However, a modified form of an income-related cost-sharing policy can be adopted. Such a policy would base the level of patients upper expense limit on income. In addition, the tax system could be used to equalize the burden of direct personal medical expenditure. Specifically the ceiling on patient liability could be determined as a fixed income share but not as a fixed dollar amount. Tax credits or refunds could be given to offset any payments that were higher than the specified income share. This policy would guarantee that the percentage of income used for paying medical bills is equal across all income classes, with the result that no family or individual would spend an inordinate amount of its resources on health-care services. Thus the prospect of extraordinary expenses resulting from prolonged illness would be equally averted by everyone, rather than inequitably by a relatively few individuals.

National Health Insurance Legislation

Perhaps the most obvious similarity among the major national health insurance bills that Congress considered during the 1970s is their emphasis on a comprehensive range of health services. All plans covered both in-hospital and out-patient services. Most provide at least limited skilled nursing home benefits and coverage of perscription drugs. Some include dental care, at least for children, and other preventive services for pregnant women and young children.[35]

The Health Security Act, proposed by Senator Edward Kennedy and supported by organized labor, was designed to reduce greatly financing based on third-party reimbursement and to shift health care financing to a per-capita and prospective budgeting basis.[36] The act would have assigned the entire financing and management of NHI to the federal government. It would have created a Health Security Board in the U.S. Department of Health and Human Services (DHHS, formerly DHEW) to administer the program. It would have levied payroll taxes and matched this amount with an equivalent sum from general revenue. The board would have established an annual national budget, not to have exceeded total receipts, and allocated it to each DHHS region on a per-capita basis in categories for institutional services, physicians' services, dental services, drugs, or appliances. Within these groups the board would then have contracted for covered services with participating providers (providers who agreed not to charge the patient for covered services).

In brief the Health Security Act would have created a system that was centrally and politically controlled, in which each participating provider received its income from the federal government.

The Health Security Act had important strengths. It recognized that the third-party-reimbursement principle provides perverse economic incentives in terms of cost containment and utilization of services. It sought to restructure health services into organized systems. Capitation financing, which it emphasized, provides incentives for economic efficiency is use of total resources. The Health Act attempted to obtain equity in terms of access and utilization of health-care resources.

The Health Security Act proposed to bring total spending under control by "top-down budgeting."[37] Top-down budgeting may indeed bring total spending under control, but without competition the budgeting mechanism has no built-in means for assuring that much useful output is produced. This weakness is especially important regarding a medical-care program whose output cannot be measured in any clear-cut way.

Finally the Health Security Act would have added over $100 billion to federal expenditures (1978 dollars), which makes it far too expensive given the size of the present budget deficit. Moreover there was no way to phase it in; it would have begun with full coverage immediately.

Universal federal third-party reimbursement was an alternative approach to national health insurance. A bill to create such a system was proposed as a legislative compromise by Senator Kennedy and Congressman Mills in 1974.[38] This is the approach adopted by the Canadian government, though their effort is a joint federal-provincial program. This system would have resulted in a program for the entire population that would have been similar to the present Medicare program. The government would have had to process over 1 billion health-insurance claims a year. If costs were to be controlled, each claim would have to be reviewed. Rules for retrospective financing would have become increasingly complex as institutions attempted to interpret them to their advantage, while the government tried to restrain cost increases.

The worst effect of universal third-party insurance would have been to destroy the incentive of consumers and physicians to reorganize the delivery system along more cost-effective lines.[39] It would have prevented consumers from having the opportunity to reap the benefit of choosing less costly systems of health care. Consumers would no longer have out-of-pocket expenses for most types of care, and larger reimbursements would have been made on their behalf if they obtained service from relatively high-cost providers.

The Kennedy–Mills bill would not have resulted in a stable equilibrium in health-care financing. The cost growth induced by the third-party-reimbursement incentives would have had to be constrained by progressively stricter government controls.

Given this situation, the government would likely have eventually been forced to place a limit on health-care spending, including negotiated prospective budgets for health-care institutions and limits on spending for physician services by state or NHI region. It is possible that within 10 years, the Kennedy–Mills bill would have become indistinguishable from the Health Security Act. The Kennedy–Mills proposal would have increased federal expenditures on health by more than $60 billion (1978 dollars).

The Comprehensive Health Insurance Plan (CHIP) proposed by the Nixon administration in 1974,[40] would have established a three-part national program including required employer-employee health-benefits programs meeting certain standards, a state-operated, "assisted health-care program" providing coverage for low-income families and for families and occupational groups who are high medical risks, and a federal program for the aged—in effect, expended Medicare.

The employee plan would have required employers to offer full-time workers a health plan that would have included hospital, medical, and preventive services, and protection against catastrophic illness. Coverage would have been implemented through private insurance and financed through employer and employee premium contributions. The assisted plan was designed to make health insurance available to all persons not otherwise insured. Many of these persons are presently receiving Medicaid. There would have been income-related deductibles, coinsurance, and a limit on each family's total health-care liability. Premiums would have been income related, and tied to the state average for the employee plan.

CHIP appealed to federal officials because most of its costs would not have been included in the federal budget. (The cost to the federal budget would have been roughly $8 billion in fiscal 1978.) Moreover it had the attractive feature of keeping much of the management and underwriting in the private sector.

However, CHIP also had some negative characteristics. It strengthened the link between job and health-plan coverage so that laid-off workers would suffer loss of coverage. Moreover, as indicated earlier, mandated employer coverage acts as a strong disincentive to hiring people with low job skills and productivity.

Another weakness of this proposal that it shared with the Kennedy–Mills bill was the mistake of considering NHI solely as a means of providing third-party reimbursement insurance coverage for the entire population instead of simultaneously viewing such legislation as providing an opportunity to develop incentives for cost control or reform of the delivery system. Thus with CHIP, cost controls would have been achieved by direct federal regulation. CHIP would not have eliminated the main barrier to competition (that most employees are offered a single health-benefit plan, usually based on third-party reimbursement). Employers would have been required to offer membership in one prepaid group practice and one individual practice association, if available, as required by the HMO Act. However, that did not consider much potential competition from health-care alliances, variable-cost insurance plans, and other innovative approaches that providers and consumers might organize to use resources wisely. Moreover CHIP would not have corrected various cost-increasing incentives in Medicare, Medicaid, and the health-expenditure subsidy created by the income tax laws. By continuing to subsidize more costly systems of care, the government would have failed to have undertaken important steps to promote competition among alternative forms of heath-care delivery.

Ultimately the need for cost controls would likely have forced the government to impose limits on spending. Within a decade or less the system that began with CHIP would likely have been similar to the Health Security Act.

A fourth alternative was known as the Long–Ribicoff proposal, named after its two senatorial sponsors, Senators Russell Long and Abraham Ribicoff.[41] If this proposal had become law, the federal government would have taken over the acute-care portion of Medicaid, providing essentially full insurance coverage for low-income families and the medically indigent. For nonpoor families, the Long–Ribicoff proposal would provide insurance against catastrophic medical expense. It would have added about $12 billion to the federal budget (1978 dollars).

The Long–Ribicoff alternative had the important strength that it targeted the available funds to those persons with the greatest need, namely the poor and medically indigent, and those with catastrophic medical expenses.

However, the plan also had important weaknesses. First, there was a major work disincentive for a low-income family at the cut-off level of income. In an economic sense there would have been little point for members of a poor family to earn more than $4,800 if they expected substantial medical bills. (This part of the legislation could have been revised so that the loss of benefits as earned income rises could be gradual in order to maintain an incentive to work.)

Another potential problem is that it locked in the concept of third-party reimbursement. Not only did this create incentives for increasing costs, but it denied to institutions that would have served the poor a predictable source of capitation financing.

Third, the Long–Ribicoff proposal would have perpetuated the third-party reimbursement system that rewards providers for cost-increasing behavior and provides no restraint on cost once the catastrophic expense limit is reached. Long–Ribicoff would have done nothing to correct the cost-increasing incentives in Medicare and the tax laws. Moreover it would not have assured every American a choice of competing plans.

Table 8–4 compares the coverage, financing, and reimbursement under the four NHI plans discussed. The Nixon proposal had the greatest number

Table 8–4
Coverage, Financing, and Type of Provider Reimbursement under Selected National Health Insurance Plans, 1975

Item	No National Health Insurance Plan	Long–Ribicoff	Nixon CHIP	Kennedy–Mills	Health Security Act (AFL-CIO)
Persons not covered by the plan (millions)	——	0	6.5	3.0	0
Direct patient payments (billions)	30.1	28.1	22.7	20.3	9.9
Sources of financing (as a percentage of total cost of plan)[a]					
Premiums	6.0	4.5	51.8	4.6	0
Federal funds	71.5	76.4	38.3	88.8	98.0
State funds	22.4	19.0	9.9	6.6	2.0
Private health-insurance business ($ billions)					
Income from sales	32.5	30.9	37.3	11.7	3.0
Administered claims and expenses	22.0	37.8	41.8	71.5	0
Extent of reimbursement of providers (in relation to total cost	——	Medicare type	Moderate	Moderate	Restricted

Source: U.S. Department of Health, Education, and Welfare, *Estimated Health Expenditures under Selected National Health Insurance Bills*, a Report to Congress, 1974.

[a] Sources of financing include payments for the plan and for Medicare and Medicaid if they are retained under the plan. Medicare and Medicaid expenditures in case there is no national health insurance, are shown under no plan.

of persons not covered by the plan and the largest contribution to financing by premiums. The Long–Ribicoff plan had the largest expenditure by patients, while the Health Security Act had the smallest contribution to patients.

Table 8–5 indicates the expenditures for the NHI plans. The most important is that even the Health Security Act only increases total health expenditures by $13 billion (1975 dollars) in comparison to no national health insurance plan.

Incremental resource costs under the Kennedy–Mills plan are $9.3 billion, compared with $6.5 billion under the Nixon plan. Since the Kennedy–Mills and Nixon plans had similar benefits for middle- and upper-income families, the greater resources available for medical care under the Kennedy–Mills plan largely reflect greater expected use of medical services by the poor and by lower-income working families.[42]

When one considers the cost of national health insurance, this usually

Table 8–5
Federal, State, and Private Expenditures for Alternative National Health Insurance Plans, 1975 *($ billions)*

Type of Expenditure	No National Health Insurance Plan	Long– Ribicoff	Nixon CHIP	Kennedy– Mills	Health Security Act (AFL-CIO)
Real resource costs	103.0	107.4	109.5	112.3	116.0
Incremental expenditures	——	4.4	6.5	9.3	13.0
Expenditures under plan					
Total	28.1	37.8	68.6	71.5	95.1
Federal	20.1	28.9	28.2	63.5	93.2
State	6.3	7.2	7.3	4.7	1.9
Private	1.7	1.7	33.1	3.3	0.0
Incremental federal expenditures					
Total	——	8.3	5.9	42.5	73.1
Programs covered by plan	——	8.8	8.1	43.4	73.1
Other programs	——	−0.5	−2.2	−0.9	0.0
Incremental state expenditures					
Total	——	0.0	−1.0	−3.7	−7.9
Programs covered by plan	——	0.9	1.0	−1.6	−4.4
Other programs	——	−0.9	−2.0	−2.1	−3.5

Source: U.S. Department of Health, Education, and Welfare *Estimated Health Expenditures under Selected National Health Insurance Bills*, Report to the Congress, 1974, pp. 25, 33, 41, 48, 61, 69, and 75.

means the amount spent by the plan. This concept of cost excludes amounts for which patients are responsible or expenditures for medical care provided by other public programs. As table 8–5 shows, expenditures for national health insurance, including any remaining parts of the Medicare and Medicaid plan, would have ranged from $38 billion under the Long–Ribicoff bill to $95 billion under the Health Security Act. This discrepancy existed primarily because the Health Security Act provided a broad range of services free of charge, whereas the Long–Ribicoff plan assumed responsibility for medical expenses only after the patient has incurred substantial costs. The total costs of the Nixon and the Kennedy–Mills plans were virtually identical under this concept of cost—$74 billion and $72 billion, respectively. This is to be expected given the similarity of benefit coverage.

Table 8–5 shows incremental federal revenues to range from $6 billion under the administration plan, to $43 billion under the Kennedy–Mills plan (and $73 billion under the Health Security Act). Additional funds for the administration plan would have been drawn from federal revenues, without specifically increasing taxes, while the Kennedy–Mills plan would have placed an additional 4 percent payroll tax on the first $20,000 of earnings and a 2.5 percent tax on self-employment income and unearned income up to a total family income of $20,000. The Kennedy–Mills plan would also have required about $8.5 billion of additional federal general revenues.

Because of the growing conservatism of the country in the 1980s and the trend toward increasing federal budget deficits, the outlook for national health insurance is bleaker than it has been for many years. The Reagan administration is seeking ways to reduce the level of federal health expenditures, and it is unlikely that there will be serious consideration to any NHI proposal during this administration. Moreover, even if a more liberal administration takes over the executive branch of the government in January 1985, the budget deficit may be too high to allow any significant consideration of national health insurance.

Summary

Health insurance is generally provided as a work-related fringe benefit that is provided on a group basis for over 80 percent of the employed population. Small firms are less likely to provide coverage than large firms, and the coverage provided by small firms is less inclusive than that provided by large firms.

The present health-insurance industry has several weaknesses: (1) It encourages hospitalization for medical conditions that could be treated on an out-patient basis. (2) Because reimbursement is frequently based on cost, it intensifies inflation in medical-care prices. (3) It makes inadequate provision for the unemployed and self-employed. Health insurance raises the demand for medical care and alters the composition of demand.

Health-maintenance organizations provide health services under a pre-paid capitation arrangement. A summary of the studies undertaken indicates that HMOs reduce both the cost and utilization of health care in comparison to conventional Blue Cross plans or commercial health insurance. However, this apparently is not done at the expense of the quality of care provided by HMOs.

Since the late 1960s a number of national health insurance plans have been introduced in Congress. The strengths, weaknesses, and estimated costs of four of them have been compared. However, the most important point regarding national health insurance is that the nation does not have such legislation in force and is unlikely to get it in the near or intermediate future.

Notes

1. Irving Pfeffer, *Insurance and Economic Theory* (Homewood, Ill.: Richard D. Irwin, 1960), pp. 45–70.

2. Robert Kaplan and Lester Lave, "Viewpoints—Patient Incentives and Hospital Insurance," *Health Services Research* 6, no. 4 (Winter 1971): 289.

3. Kenneth Arrow, "Uncertainty and the Welfare Economics of Medical Care," *American Economic Review* 53, no. 5 (December 1963): 941.

4. M. Pachl, "Use of Hospitals by Blue Cross Members in 1968," *Blue Cross Reports*, Research Series 3, December 1969, p. 91.

5. Arrow, "Uncertainty and the Welfare Economics of Medical Care," p. 941.

6. See, for example, A. Donabedian, "An Evaluation of Prepaid Group Practice," *Inquiry* 6, no. 3 (September 1969): 3; Paul Densen, Sam Shapiro, Ellen Jones, and Irving Baldinger, "Prepaid Medical Care and Hospital Utilization," *Hospitals* 36, no. 22 (November 16, 1962): 63; P. Hardwick and H. Wolfe, "A Multifaceted Approach to Incentive Reimbursement," *Medical Care* 8, no. 3 (May–June 1970): 173.

7. Mark Pauly, "Health Insurance and Hospital Behavior," in Colton Lindsay (Ed.), *New Directions in Public Health Care: An Evaluation of Proposals for National Health Insurance* (San Francisco, Calif.: Institute for Contemporary Studies, 1976), p. 107.

8. Ibid., p. 108.

9. Ibid., p. 111.

10. Joseph Newhouse, Charles Phelps, and William Schwartz, "Policy Options and the Impact of National Health Insurance," *New England*

Journal of Medicine 290, no. 24 (June 13, 1974): 1345–1359.

11. Martin Feldstein, "The Welfare Loss of Excess Health Insurance," *Journal of Political Economy* 81, no. 2 (March–April 1973): 252.

12. Alain Enthoven, "Consumer-Choice Health Plan, Part I," *New England Journal of Medicine* 298, no. 12 (March 23, 1978): 653.

13. Judith Feder, Jack Hadley, and John Holahan, *Insuring the Nation's Health: Market Competition, Catastrophic and Comprehensive Approaches* (Washington, D.C.: Urban Institute Press, 1981), p. 13.

14. Suresh Malhotra, Kenneth McCaffree, John Wills, and Jean Baker, *Employment-Related Health Benefits: A Survey of Establishments in the Private Nonfarm Sector*, Final Report, vol. 2 (Seattle, Wash.: Battelle Human Affairs Research Center, 1980), tables 1 and 2, pp. 24 and 25.

15. Ibid., tables 2 and 3, pp. 29 and 30.

16. Dorothy Kittner, "Changes in Health Plans Reflect Broader Coverage," *Monthly Labor Review* 101, no. 9 (September 1978): 57–59.

17. Marjorie Smith Carroll and Ross Arnett, "Private Health Insurance Plans in 1977: Coverage, Enrollment, and Financial Experience," *Health Care Financing Review* I, no.2 (Fall 1979): 22.

18. Department of Health and Human Services, Social Security Administration Publication no. 05-10050 *Your Medicare Handbook* (Washington, D.C.: U.S. Government Printing Office, April 1982), p. 46.

19. Harold Luft, "Assessing the Evidence on HMO Performance," *Milbank Memorial Fund Quarterly* 58, no. 4 (Fall 1980): 503.

20. Ibid., p. 504.

21. R.P. Wersinger and A. Sorenson, "An Analysis of the Health Status and Cost Experience of an HMO Population Compared with a Blue Cross/Blue Shield Matched Control Group," University of Rochester, New York, 1980 (mimeographed).

22. Luft, Evidence on HMO Performance," p. 511–512.

23. W.E. McAuliffe, "Measuring the Quality of Medical Care: Process Versus Outcome," *Milbank Memorial Fund Quarterly* 57, no. 1 (Winter 1979): 118–152.

24. S. Shapiro, L. Weiner, and P. Densen, "Comparison of Prematurity and Perinatal Mortality in a General Population and in the Population of a Prepaid Group Practice Medical Care Plan," *American Journal of Public Health* 48, no. 2 (February 1958): 170–185.

25. F.C. Cunningham and J.W. Williamson, "How Does the Quality of Health Care in HMOs Compare to That in Other Settings? An Analytic Literature Review," *Group Health Journal* 1, no. 2 (Winter 1980): 4–25.

26. Isadore S. Falk, "National Health Insurance for the United States," *Public Health Reports* 92, no. 5 (September–October 1977): 399.

27. O.W. Anderson, *The Uneasy Equilibrium: Private and Public Fi-*

nancing of the United States, 1875–1965 (New Haven, Conn.: College and University Press, 1968), pp. 69–75.

28. Falk, "National Health Insurance for the United States," p. 401.

29. Ibid., p. 402.

30. Rachel Boaz, "Equity in Paying Health Care Services under a National Insurance System," *Milbank Memorial Fund Quarterly/Health and Society* 53, no. 3 (Summer 1975): 338.

31. Ibid., pp. 339–340.

32. Ibid., p. 343.

33. Newhouse, Phelps, and Schwartz, "Policy Options and the Impact of National Health Insurance," p. 1346.

34. Charles Phelps and Joseph Newhouse, "Effects of Coinsurance on the Use of Physician Services," *Social Security Bulletin* 35, no. 6 (June 1977): 10, 16–17.

35. Karen Davis, *National Health Insurance: Benefits, Costs and Consequences* (Washington, D.C.: The Brookings Institution, 1975), pp. 110–111.

36. Health Security Act, S.3, 95th Cong., 1st sess., January 10, 1977.

37. Enthoven, p. 656.

38. Comprehensive National Health Insurance Act of 1974, S.3286, 93rd Cong., 2nd sess., April 2, 1974.

39. E. Vayda, "Prepaid Group Practice under Universal Health Insurance in Canada," *Medical Care* 15, no. 5 (1977): 382–389.

40. Comprehensive Health Insurance Act of 1974, S.2970, 93rd Cong., 2nd sess., February 6, 1974.

41. Catastrophic Health and Medical Assistance Reform Act of 1975, S.2470, 94th Cong., 1st sess., September 11, 1975.

42. Davis, *National Health Insurance*, pp. 132–133.

9   Health and Poverty

This chapter considers the two-way relationship between low income and health status. The association between income and mortality, morbidity, and the utilization of health and dental services are explored. Medicaid, the major health program for the poor and medically indigent, is examined. Finally, some discussion is presented regarding health services for American Indians.

The official definition of poverty income was developed by the Bureau of the Census. According to that agency the poverty-level income cutoff (the maximum amount of income one can receive and still be in poverty) is three times the amount of money required to purchase an economy food plan.[1] This plan, established by the U.S. Department of Agriculture in 1961, is based on a basket of food items required for a minimally adequate diet. Changes in the prices of these items (usually upward) result in a movement of the poverty income cutoff. Since the economy food plan varies depending on family size, family composition, sex, and age of the family head, as well as residence (farm or nonfarm), the poverty income cutoff also differs according to these socioeconomic characteristics.

In estimating the number of persons below the poverty income level, the Bureau of the Census includes total earnings from wages and salaries, self-employment income, Social Security payments, public-assistance payments, property income in the form of dividends, interest, or rent, unemployment and workmen's compensation, government and private employee pensions, and other income. It does not include the imputed monetary value of in-kind transfer programs such as food stamps, medical care, or housing assistance.

In 1979 the poverty level varied from $3,855 for a single person, to an average of $12,322 for a two-parent, nonfarm family, with six or more children.[2] Table 9–1 indicates the trend in the poverty-income threshold from 1960 to 1980 for a nonfarm family of four. In 1960 the poverty-income threshold was set at approximately $3,000; by 1980 it had increased to $8,414.

From 1960 to 1969 there was a fairly dramatic reduction in the absolute and relative incidence of poverty: from almost 40 million people (22 percent of the civilian population), to 24 million (12 percent). During the latter half of this period, unemployment was very low, partly because of the economic impact of the war in Vietnam. From 1969 to 1979 the number of people

Table 9–1
Trends in Poverty-Income Threshold, Consumer Price Index, and Poverty Population 1960–1980

Year	Poverty-Income Threshold (current dollars)[a]	Consumer Price Index 1972 = 100	Poverty Population	
			Millions	As Percentage of Total Civilian Population
1960	3,022	70.8	39.6	22.4
1961	3,054	71.5	39.6	21.9
1962	3,089	72.3	38.6	21.0
1963	3,128	73.2	36.4	19.5
1964	3,169	74.1	36.1	19.1
1965	3,223	75.4	33.2	17.3
1966	3.317	77.6	28.5	14.2
1967	3,410	79.8	27.8	14.2
1968	3,553	83.2	25.4	12.8
1969	3,743	87.6	24.1	12.1
1970	3,968	92.8	25.4	12.6
1971	4,137	96.8	25.6	12.5
1972	4,275	100.0	24.5	11.9
1973	4,540	108.4	23.0	11.1
1974	5,038	116.1	23.4	11.2
1975	5,500	123.4	25.9	12.3
1976	5,815	134.6	25.0	11.8
1977	6,191	144.0	24.7	11.6
1978	6,662	158.7	24.5	11.4
1979	7,412	176.9	26.1	11.7
1980	8,414	200.8	29.3	13.0

Source: U.S. Department of Commerce, *Statistical Abstract, 1982–83* (Washington, D.C.: U.S. Government Printing Office, 1982), p. 440–441.

a. For a nonfarm family of four persons.

with incomes below the poverty level remained approximately the same. However, in 1980 there was a sharp increase in the number of persons living in poverty, because the combination of inflation and recession.

There is evidence that many of those who remained poor throughout this period probably have serious disabling conditions. As poverty has declined, the average level of health of the poor may have worsened because relatively healthier people experienced sufficient gains in income to be above the poverty-income cutoff.

In 1980 over one-third of the poor were children under age 18. Thirteen percent were 65 or over, the group most likely to be covered by both the Medicare and Medicaid programs. Two-thirds of the poor are white, and 40 percent reside in nonmetropolitan areas. Low-income persons are concentrated disproportionately in the South, which has 31 percent of the total population but 44 percent of the poor and 60 percent of the poor nonmetropolitan residents. Medicaid, a combined federal and state health program for the poor and medically indigent, is much more limited in terms of coverage in Southern states and rural areas so that many of the poor who live in these locations do not receive adequate health services.[3]

The structure of poor families is important in the case of Medicaid, which bases eligibility, to some extent, on the presence of children and the absence of a father in the family. Half the states participating in Medicaid do not cover nonelderly two-parent families; the others do not cover two-parent families unless the father is unemployed and not receiving unemployment compensation.

There are several reasons why the health care of the low-income population is an important public policy matter. One reason is that improving health-care services to the poor causes them to experience a gain in productivity and personal development. Thus one argument for a major governmental role in providing health-care services for the poor is that it is an investment in human capital that the poor will not make without government assistance. It is widely accepted that poor health results in relatively low incomes. In some cases those living in poverty are disadvantaged from an early age because of inadequate care and nutrition during pregnancy and infancy. There is some evidence that malnutrition not only reduces physical growth and development, but mental capacity as well. Limited by various conditions, many of the poor are unable to lead normally healthy, productive lives. Investment in health and nutrition programs may have a high social return that manifests itself in a more equitable distribution of income, reduced economic dependency, and higher productivity and output.[4]

A second reason for concern is purely humanitarian considerations.[5] Unlike the human-investment factor which maintains that better health will result in higher productivity and income for the poor, the former reason has no economic rationale. It simply maintains that no one should suffer needlessly from ill health or die because of lack of money to obtain adequate nutrition or medical care.

A major role for the federal government in providing the poor with health care results from the numerous failures of the private market. Thus merely guaranteeing the poor a minimum level of income is unlikely to result in adequate health levels unless that minimum income level is set at a very high figure—something that is not politically feasible.

For example, a guaranteed income level might be sufficient to cover health-care needs as well as other basic goods and services if the low-income persons were able to purchase health or accident insurance. Unfortunately, however, private companies do not furnish this protection at a cost many poor people can afford. In addition, these firms have been reluctant to market comprehensive policies for the elderly because of concern about the proportion of high-risk policyholders who could not be screened effectively by physical examination. The insurance policies that are available have limited coverage, exclude preexisting conditions, seldom cover nursing home care if infirmity or senility occurs, and are generally inadequate to protect older people and their children from the high out-of-pocket costs of catastrophic illness.

The nonelderly poor are in a similar circumstance. Persons who are not employed cannot participate in group employment policies with relatively low premium rates. Private companies generally do not provide comprehensive health-insurance policies for the poor, who, partly because of their numerous medical conditions, are considered a high risk. The few policies available are usually limited in benefits and require a high premium, particularly in relation to the individual's income. Moreover, frequently provisions are included in policies that permit companies the option of dropping coverage should the beneficiary become a poor risk. For the disabled low-income person or those with definite health problems, companies are simply unwilling to provide coverage.

Other failures of the private market also suggest a larger role for government. Communities characterized by poverty or racial discrimination generally are plagued by shortages of health labor power and health facilities. Insurance, whether publicly provided or publicly subsidized, can do little in the short run to ameliorate these shortages. Physicians, attracted by the high incomes the can be earned in the suburbs, have been leaving central cities and rural areas for some time. Only a relatively small number of students from minority groups are currently enrolled in medical and other health professional schools and many of these will practice in more affluent areas upon completion of studies. Partly as a result, these is a scarcity of health professionals willing to work in areas inhabited by a high proportion of minority and low-income persons.[6]

Income and Mortality

Several studies have documented the fact that persons with low income and limited schooling have higher death rates than others.[7] A 1962–63 study of death rates by age, sex, and family income in the year before death, showed that death rates of males and females under 55 were from four to ten times higher than those with family incomes below $2,000 as compared to those with family incomes above $8,000.[8] Part of the difference might have occured because people with long illnesses may have had abnormally low incomes in the year preceding death. However, this seems less likely to explain high death rates among low-income younger women, since family income at that time was not highly dependent on the earnings and therefore health of female family members.

Kitagawa and Hauser found that age-adjusted mortality rates were 80 percent higher for white male family members 25 to 64 years old with family incomes under $2,000 than for males in the same age classification with family incomes of $10,000 or more. For white female family members, the mortality rate was 40 percent higher in the lowest family-income class than in the highest.[9]

Kitagawa and Hauser also compared death rates by cause with educational levels (without holding income constant). They found that in 1960, for white males 25 years old and over, those with less than 8 years of education had higher death rates than those with 1 year or more of college from the following causes: tuberculosis (300 percent higher), diabetes mellitus (25 percent higher), cerebrovascular diseases (24 percent higher), hypertensive diseases (23 percent higher), influenza and pneumonia (60 percent higher), accidents (71 percent higher), and suicide (87 percent higher). However, college-educated white males had higher age-adjusted death rates than white males with less than 8 years of education for malignant neoplasm of the prostate (95 percent) and cirrhosis of the liver (6 percent). Death rates did not differ by years of schooling for cardiovascular and renal diseases. Among white women, those with a college education tended to have lower death rates than less-educated women for the same diseases as the men with the exception of malignant neoplasms of the breast, where death rates were 42 percent higher for college-educated women as compared to women with 8 years or less of schooling. Regarding cirrhosis of the liver, death rates did not vary appreciably by years of schooling.[10]

Among both whites and nonwhites, infant mortality rates tend to decrease as income rises.[11] However, the relationship is imperfect. For both races the lowest infant death rates occur at the middle-income level, with very high rates at lower-income-levels, and lower rates at high-income levels. Infant mortality among white families with incomes of $10,000 is 29.7 percent lower than among white families with incomes under $3,000; while infant mortality among nonwhite families with incomes of $10,000 is only 11.5 percent lower than that of nonwhite families with incomes of under $3,000. Also, white infant mortality appears to be related to the father's education in that the rate is 37.7 percent lower in families in which the father's education is 1 to 3 years of college, compared with the rate in families in which the father's level of education is eighth grade or less. However, nonwhite infant mortality is only 11.3 percent lower in families at the higher educational level.[12]

An explanation for the weaker relationship between infant mortality and income and education among nonwhites is that the health of the mother and the outcome of her pregnancy is influenced more by the environment in which she was reared than by her present environment.

Causes of infant deaths that are more prevalent in low-income families are infectious and parasitic diseases, influenza, pneumonia and other re-spiratory diseases, accidents, and various diseases of the digestive system. Babies are most vulnerable to these conditions when they have just been discharged from the hospital and taken home. Improper sterilization of bottles, impure water, or unsafe sanitation may cause diarrhea, which in some cases may lead to severe dehydration, hospitalization, and death. Poor housing with crowding, and inadequate heating and ventilation, can in-crease the incidence of respiratory illness. Most of the conditions named can be treated effectively if the infant receives prompt medical attention. Delay in seeking medical care tends to be more common among low-income families.[13]

The effect of low income on infant mortality can also be discerned when trends in infant mortality rates are compared by states. In 1965 the infant mortality rate in the ten states with the highest rates of poverty was 29.5 death per 1,000 live births, 1.3 times that of the ten states with the lowest rates of poverty. Between 1965 and 1974 infant mortality declined more rapidly in the ten highest poverty states than in most of the other states, reducing this ratio to 1.19 by 1974. In 1969–1971 the life expectancy in the states with the lowest incidence of poverty was 3–4 percent greater than in those states with the highest incidence of poverty.[14]

As indicated in table 9–2, the prevalence of chronic conditions is closely linked to family income. Among persons 17 to 44 years of age, those in the lowest-income classification experience prevalence rates 15–30 percent higher than those in the highest-income classification. For older persons the effect of income on prevalence of chronic conditions is much greater.

There is little evidence of any reduction in the incidence of long-term chronic health problems from 1964 to 1972. For people between 45 and 64, the prevalence of chronic conditions such as arthirtis, diabetes, hearing and visual impariments, heart conditions, and hypertension, remains two to three times higher for those with low incomes than for others.

It would be inappropriate to conclude, however, that medical-care programs for the poor have had no impact on the prevalence of chronic conditions. As the death rate declines, the incidence of chronic conditions can be expected to increase. Thus the relative stability in the prevalence rates for these conditions during a period when the death rate declined should be little cause for concern.

Improved medical care moreover can be expected to reduce the preva-lence of chronic conditions only after a considerable period of time. For those who already have one or more of the chronic conditions enumerated in table 9–2, medical care can do little to remove the condition. However, for many of those with chronic conditions, greater access to medical care can mean the relief of pain and suffering with the concomitant ability to function more effectively.

Table 9–2
Prevalence of Selected Chronic Conditions, by Family Income, 1968–1973, by Age, Number per 1,000 Persons

17–44 Years

Family Income	Arthritis	Asthma	Diabetes	Heart Conditions	Hypertension	Hearing Impairment	Vision Impairment
				Disease or Condition			
Under $5,000	46.9	34.1	11.4	32.5	48.9	55.4	43.2
$5,000–$10,000	40.5	23.6	8.7	23.3	40.8	44.0	31.7
$10,000–$15,000	38.7	24.4	8.4	22.5	35.9	39.8	28.7
$15,000 and over	35.9	26.8	8.0	24.3	29.8	35.8	30.9

45–64 Years

Family Income	Arthritis	Asthma	Diabetes	Heart Conditions	Hypertension	Hearing Impairment	Vision Impairment
				Disease or Condition			
Under $5,000	297.8	53.5	74.1	139.3	172.7	158.9	114.1
$5,000–$10,000	200.3	33.5	43.8	92.5	125.4	118.1	57.4
$10,000–$15,000	163.7	23.7	37.8	74.3	121.3	107.3	45.9
$15,000 and over	159.8	22.7	30.5	66.6	105.3	85.9	48.9

Source: U.S. Public Health Service, Health Resources Administration, *Health: United States, 1975*, DHEW Publication no. 76-1232, (Washington, D.C.: U.S. Government Printing Office, 1976), pp. 481 and 487.

While the information on trends in the prevalence of chronic conditions indicate little change, there are some modest improvements. The aged, poor or not, experienced a reduction in limitation of activity caused by chronic conditions. Moreover, although children as a whole experienced slightly increased limitation of activity, poor children showed a smaller gain than other children.

Table 9–3 indicates the degree of chronic activity limitation by income. The fact that over 30 percent of those with incomes under $3,000 a year experienced some limitation of activity contrasted with the fact that less than 10 percent of those earning $25,000 or more experienced some activity limitation. However, information such as this does not indicate whether low income ultimately results in activity limitation or whether it is the other way around.

Use of Medical Care

One of the most significant changes in utilization to occur between 1964 and 1974 was the greater use of medical care services by low-income people. The poor have always had greater morbidity than other Americans but generally have obtained less treatment from physicians. The 1964–1974 period was one in which this historical pattern was reversed, so that by the end of the period the poor had more visits to physicians than the nonpoor. (See table 9–4.) To a lesser extent the poor also made greater use of dental services. The percentage of those with incomes under $5,000 who saw a dentist rose from 29 percent in 1970 to 34 percent in 1974, while the proportion of

Table 9–3
Percentage Distribution of Persons by Degree of Activity Limitation and Income

Income	All Persons	With No Limitation of Activity	With Limitation but Not in Major Activity	With Limitation in Amount or Kind of Major Activity	Unable to Carry on Major Activity
Under $3,000	100	69.8	5.1	16.1	9.0
$3,000–$5,000	100	72.8	4.3	13.6	9.2
$5,000–$7,000	100	79.9	3.9	10.2	6.0
$7,000–$10,000	100	85.5	3.5	7.4	3.6
$10,000–$14,000	100	89.8	3.2	5.3	1.7
$15,000–$25,000	100	91.2	3.1	4.6	1.2
$25,000+	100	91.4	3.6	4.1	0.9

Source: U.S. Public Health Service, National Center for Health Statistics, "Health Interview Survey," unpublished data.

Table 9–4
Physician Visits per Person, by Family Income, 1964, 1970, and 1974

1964	Number of Visits	1970	Number of Visits	1974	Number of Visits
All incomes	4.5	All incomes	4.6	All incomes	4.9
Under $4,000	4.3	Under $2,000	5.3	Under $2,000	5.9
$4,000–$6,999	4.5	$2,000–$3,999	5.1	$2,000–$3,999	5.3
$7,000–$9,999	4.7	$4,000–$6,999	4.4	$4,000–$6,999	5.0
$10,000 and over	5.1	$7,000–$9,999	4.3	$7,000–$9,999	5.1
Ration of highest	1.19	$10,000–$14,999	4.6	$10,000–$14,999	4.6
to lowest		$15,000 and over	4.9	$15,000 and over	4.9
		Ratio of highest	.94	Ratio of highest	.84
		to lowest		to lowest	

Source: U.S. Department of Health, Education, and Welfare, National Center for Health Statistics, "Volume of Physician Visits by Place of Visit and Type of Service, United States, July 1963–June 1964, Vital and Health Statistics, Series 10, no. 18 (Washington, D.C.: U.S. Government Printing Office, 1965), pp. 18–19 and 29; Melvin Rudov and Nancy Santangelo, *Health Status of Minorities and Low-Income Groups,* DHEW Publication no. (HRA)79-627 (Washington, D.C.: U.S. Government Printing Office, 1979) pp. 238–239.

higher-income people seeing a dentist declined. The hospitalization rate for the same group increased by 40 percent from 1964 to 1974, far surpassing that of other income classes.

Increases in visits to physicians may occur either because more people go to see physicians or because those who do, go more frequently, or both. The proportion of the poor seeing a physician over a 2 year interval rose: in 1964, 28 percent had not seen a physician for 2 years or more; by 1978 this percentage was only 14. Progress was considerable among poor children, one-third of whom had not seen a physician for 2 years or more in 1964. By 1978 this figure had declined to 13 percent. Despite this gain, poor children were still 29 percent less likely to have seen a physician in the 2 years before 1978 than nonpoor children.[15]

Most of the federal health programs of the past decade have been primarily concerned with medical care, but some programs also include dental services. Most of the comprehensive health centers provide routine dental care. The federal Medicaid program covers dental care as an optional service, and most states have elected to extend at least some dental services to Medicaid recipients.

The dental health of the poor has been inadequate for many years. In 1971 low-income adults between the ages of 45 and 64 were almost three times as likely to have lost all their own teeth as were adults of the same age with incomes above $15,000. Among the aged, almost 60 percent of those with incomes below $3,000 had lost their teeth; but only 35 percent of those with incomes above $15,000 had lost them.[16]

Poor dental health is evident in childhood. From 1963 to 1965 among children between 6 and 11 years of age, those from poor families had an average of 3.4 decayed teeth; but children from nonpoor families had an average of only 2.0 decayed teeth. Nearly twice as many poor children as nonpoor children between 12 and 17 had decayed or missing permanent teeth.[17] By 1971–1974 the situation had shown only slight improvement for children aged 12 to 17, but the number of decayed teeth for 6- to 11-year-olds from poor families fell to 2.5, compared to 1.8 decayed teeth for nonpoor children of the same age.[18]

Although the dental health of the poor remains at substandard levels, there was an increase in their utilization of dental services from 1964 to 1978. In 1964 62.5 percent of the poor had not seen a dentist in the past 2 years compared with 40.9 percent of the nonpoor. By 1978 these percentages were reduced to 49.4 and 33.3, respectively.

For poor children, the average annual number of dental visits increased from 0.5 to almost one visit per child. Despite this about 52 percent of poor children had not seen a dentist in the 2 years before 1978.[19]

Because the poor are afflicted with more chronic conditions than others (see table 9–2), and because their health problems are generally more severe, it is not surprising that low-income people are hospitalized more than others. The period 1964–1973 was characterized by a major gain in the number of low-income people receiving hospital care. Thus in 1964 discharges from short-stay hospitals averaged 14 for every 100 low-income people; by 1973 this had risen to 24 per 100 people, a 70 percent increase over the period. At the same time there was only a modest increase in the hospitalization rates of higher-income persons.[20]

A major increase in the hospitalization rate also occurred for older people. In 1964 there were 19 hospital discharges for every 100 people 65 or over. However, this had increased to 35 discharges in 1973.

Among surgical operations there was a general increase the the total population from 1963–1965 to 1976–1978. However, the proportional increase for the poor was considerably greater than the nonpoor for all age groups. (See table 9–5.)

Even though the poor as a whole receive more care from physicians than formerly, major differences do remain in the setting, continuity, and type of health care available to low-income persons. In 1974 almost 27 percent of families earning less than $5,000, but 15 percent of families earning over $15,000 had no "usual" place for obtaining care. Eight percent of the low-income families used hospital emergency rooms as sources of care, while only 2 percent of those earning over $15,000 used hospital emergency rooms regularly. Care is usually more inconvenient to obtain for the poor.[21] They spend 58 percent more time than those with higher incomes traveling and waiting to see a physician.

Table 9–5
Rates of Surgery per 1,000 Persons, Poor and Nonpoor, by Age, 1963–1965 and 1978–1978

	1963–1965			*1976–1978*	
Age	*Poor*	*Nonpoor*	*Age*	*Poor*	*Nonpoor*
Under 15	20.1	34.3	Under 15	26.6	31.0
15–44	47.5	52.5	15–44	66.4	55.9
45–64	52.9	68.8	45–64	86.1	78.6
65+	57.9	72.1	65+	105.1	105.3

Source: U.S. Department of Health and Human Services, *Health: United States, 1980*, DHHS Publication no. (PHS)81-1232 (Washington, D.C.: U.S. Government Printing Office, December 1980), pp. 52–54.

Poor Health as a Cause of Low Income

There is a substantial evidence that many persons live at poverty level incomes because of poor health. For instance, among men between the ages of 25 and 59, not in the labor force in March 1968, 51.9 percent of the whites and 62.9 percent of the blacks list health as the cause.[22] Parnes indicates that among white men whose health limited the kind of work they could undertake, their unemployment rate was 140 percent higher than for those white males with no health limitations. The unemployment differences for blacks (with health limitations as compared to without) was 90 percent.[23]

Luft (using data on 1967 earnings) measured the impact of disability on income for each of the race-sex categories. The income loss per sick adult is indicated below:[24]

Black men	$1,716
White men	2,208
White women	863
Black women	1,479

Based on these data, the average disabled black women suffers an earnings loss equal to 37.8 percent of her yearly earnings; while a white man loses 35.8 percent of his earnings. However, the greatest loss is suffered by black males, whose income declines 45 percent after incurring a disability.

Poor health apparently has different effects on each group. Black men are much more likely to drop out of the labor force or work fewer weeks than white men, while the latter receive larger declines in hourly wages and earnings. For women, the impacts by race are similar. Thus black women are more likely to drop out and reduce their hours per week, while white women have a larger loss in wage rates and overall earnings.

Given the different educational backgrounds and jobs open to blacks and whites at the time the data were collected, the following description of the impact of poor health seems likely. Whites, because of their higher education and earnings, are able to shift to other jobs that one can perform even if disabled. This job change is accompanied, on average, by a substantial decline in hourly wages and, thus, yearly earnings. Blacks did not have the range of jobs open to them as did whites. The lower educational attainment of the former and job discrimination make other positions hard to get. The hourly wage of blacks could not fall too much because it was close to the minimum even for healthy blacks. Since they were at the bottom of the wage scale, blacks could not trade off income reductions for less painful or arduous work. Blacks, therefore, were more likely to be forced out of the labor force if they became disabled.[25]

A number of studies have indicated the decline in income that occurs after one becomes ill. For example, a study based on a sample of Social Security disability applicants in New Orleans, Minneapolis-St. Paul, and Columbus, Ohio areas who were not institutionalized, indicated that median income fell from $482 to $220 per month after disability.[26] An earlier investigation concerned a 20-year follow-up survey of Hagerstown, Maryland families. No families suffered a reduction in socioeconomic status if they were well at the beginning and end of the period; while 9.2 percent of the families that had an illness in 1943, after being free of illness in 1923, had a reduction in socioeconomic status.[27]

Medicaid

Medicaid is a combined federal and state program. Administrative responsibility and roughly half the costs are absorbed by state and local governments. Medicaid provides a wide range of medical services to those on welfare and to some of the medically indigent (persons whose incomes are too low to pay for medical care).

The Social Security Amendments of 1950 provided federal matching funds for medical payments to hospitals, physicians, and other providers of medical care on behalf of those receiving public assistance. By 1960 about forty states were participating in this effort, with medical care expenditures reaching $0.5 billion.

The Social Security Amendments of 1960, known as the Kerr–Mills Act, greatly expanded federal assistance for health care. The proportion of federal funds was increased and coverage was provided to the medically indigent elderly who did not require cash assistance.

In 1965 Medicaid replaced the Kerr–Mills Act and thus increased the level of benefits, as well as their scope. The new legislation also tried to impose more uniformity on state programs. However, Medicaid did follow many of the general principles of previous welfare-related programs of medical assistance for the poor. It maintained a joint federal-state responsibility, with federal matching funds and broad, federally established minimum requirements for state programs. In addition, state governments were given administrative responsibility and discretion to set eligibility standards and benefit coverage as long as these were consistent with state guidelines.[28]

Medicaid expanded and improved the existing program of medical care for the poor and aged. It increased the federal share which, in 1980, ranged from 50 to 78 percent of the total depending inversely on a state's per-capita income—that is, the smaller the state's per-capita income, the larger the federal share. Medicaid specified a mandatory set of medical services that each state had to provide, as well as an optional set of services for which some federal assistance in funding was available.

Participation in Medicaid is linked to eligibility for welfare, and Medicaid thus shares the complexity of the welfare system. States are required to cover all families participating in the Aid to Families with Dependent Children (AFDC) Program. States may also cover all blind, aged, and disabled recipients of Supplemental Security Income (SSI) or they may limit coverage to SSI recipients meeting the more restrictive state Medicaid eligibility requirements of January 1, 1972 (before the implementation of SSI). All thirty-five states have elected to cover all SSI recipients.

In addition to covering cash-assistance recipients, states may provide Medicaid coverage to the medically needy; that is persons whose income is too low to pay substantial medical expenses. Twenty-eight states extend coverage to the medically needy.

AFDC is limited in a majority of states to families without a father residing in the home. Twenty-four states and two jurisdictions also extend AFDC and Medicaid coverage to families with unemployed fathers who are not recieving unemployment compensation. Seventeen states and three jurisdictions cover all children in families with incomes below AFDC eligibility level, regardless of the employment status of the parents or the family composition.

States covering the medically needy establish income, asset, and family-composition tests similar to those for public assistance recipients. Medically needy income levels for a family of four as of December 1980, ranged from $3,100 in Arkansas to $6,900 in Rhode Island.[29] Families with incomes above these levels may also be eligible if their incomes are below this amount after deducting medical expenses incurred (the so-called spend-down provision).

As a result of this complex set of eligibility requirements, the following low-income persons are not eligible for Medicaid assistance;

1. Widows and other single persons under 65 and childless couples;
2. Most two-parent families (which constitute 70 percent of the rural poor and almost half the poor families in metropolitan areas);
3. Families with a father working at a marginal, low-paying job;
4. Families with an unemployed father in the 26 states that do not extend welfare payments to this group, and unemployed fathers receiving unemployment compensation in other states;
5. Medically needy families that do not voluntarily provide this additional coverage;
6. Single women pregnant with their first child in the 20 states that do not provide welfare aid or eligibility for the "unborn child";
7. Children of poor families not receiving AFDC in the 33 states that do not take advantage of the optional Medicaid category called "all needy children under 21."[30]

In 1979 an estimated 21.5 million people received services covered by Medicaid. This number was slightly below the size of the poverty population, which was estimated at 25 million that year. The Council of Economic Advisors estimated that 30 percent of all Medicaid recipients had incomes above the poverty level in 1973.[31] If that proportion has remained constant over time, this suggests that only 18 million people, or 70 percent of the poor, were covered by Medicaid in 1979 and that approximately 7 million poor people were excluded.

Medicaid Costs

The cost of the Medicaid program has increased rapidly. Combined federal and state-local expenditures increased from $3.5 billion in 1968 to 20.5 billion in fiscal 1979. (See table 9–6.)

Three factors explain almost all the increase in expenditures. These are the increase in the number of Medicaid recipients covered under the AFDC program; sustained medical-care price inflation; and the high cost of skilled nursing facilities and intermediate-care facilities for the aged poor and disabled. Expenditures for these two items more than doubled between 1973 and 1979.

The rapid growth in the number receiving welfare payments in the late 1960s and early 1970s accounted for a large portion of the increased cost of Medicaid. Between 1968 and 1972 the total number of Medicaid recipients rose by 70 percent. Since the economy was relatively prosperous at that time, most of the increase was due to the increased number of eligible people

Table 9–6
Number of Recipients, Total Payments, and Payment per Recipient Under Medicaid, Fiscal Years 1968–1979

Fiscal Year	Number of Recipients (millions	Total Federal and State Payments ($ billions)	Payments per Recipient ($)	Medical-Care Price Index 1968 = 100	Payments per Recipient (1968 $)
1968	11.5	3.45	300	100.0	300
1969	12.1	4.35	361	106.9	338
1970	14.5	4.09	351	113.7	309
1971	18.0	6.35	353	121.0	292
1972	18.0	7.35	408	124.9	327
1973	19.6	8.64	440	129.8	329
1974	21.1	10.0	471	141.8	323
1975	22.2	12.3	554	158.9	348
1976	22.9	14.1	615	173.9	353
1977	22.9	16.3	710	192.9	368
1978	22.2	18.0	810	207.8	390
1979	21.5	20.5	951	228.0	417

Source: U.S. Department of Health, Education, and Welfare, Health Care Financing Administration, *Data on the Medicaid Program: Eligibility, Services, Expenditures, Fiscal Years 1966–1977* (Washington, D.C.: Institute for Medicaid Management, 1977), p. 34; and Donald Muse and Darwin Sawyer, *The Medicare and Medicaid Data Book, 1981* (Washington, D.C.: U.S. Department of Health and Human Services, 1982), pp. 13 and 20.

applying for benefits. Estimates indicate that the percentage of eligible people participating in AFDC increased from 60 percent to more than 90 percent.[32]

The second major factor has been the sustained inflation in medical-care prices. After the removal of wage and price controls on the health industry in April 1974, the medical-care index rose at an annual rate of 13 percent—in sharp contrast with the rate of 4 percent when the economic stabilization program was in effect.[33] Hospital costs went up at the even faster annual rate of 16 percent. From 1975 to 1979 medical-care prices rose an average of 9 percent, with the prices of hospital services increasing 11 percent. These higher prices were reflected in Medicaid expenditures.

Annual Medicaid payments per recipient in constant 1968 "medical dollars" (expenditures divided by the medical-care price index) averaged $417 per person in fiscal 1979, as against $338 in 1969 (table 9–4). Thus, from 1969 to 1977, almost all of the growth in Medicaid costs could be traced to the rise in medical-care prices and to the increased number of people receiving services. On the average, Medicaid beneficiaries in 1977 were receiving approximately the same real services as in the early years of the program. Since 1977 the number of beneficiaries has fallen as some states have increased eligibility restrictions. The rapid rise in expenditures has outstripped the rise in prices, and payments per recipient have increased sharply.

Finally, the third source of expenditure increases under Medicaid is the high cost of institutionalization for the elderly poor and disabled population that is unable to carry out normal daily activities without nursing assistance. The aged are the only sizable group for which there has been any substantial increase in constant dollar expenditures in recent years. The increase was at least 30 percent between 1968 and 1979. The tendency to place large numbers of the elderly in nursing homes—where average Medicaid expenditures were $5,500 a person in 1979—accounts for a major portion of Medicaid costs. Thirty-five percent of all Medicaid payments, amounting to $7 billion in fiscal 1979, is spent for services provided by nursing homes and intermediate-care facilities. Sixty percent of Medicaid expenditures is for services to aged or disabled adults.[34]

Medical-Care Utilization under Medicaid

One approach to assessing the contribution of Medicaid to health services is to compare the use of medical services by Medicaid recipients with that of other low-income persons. In order to facilitate this comparison, an econometric analysis of the use of hospital and physicians' services by recipients of public assistance and by other low-income persons was conducted by Davis and Reynolds.[35] Receipt of public assistance was used as a crude proxy for Medicaid eligibility.

The major findings of the study are presented in table 9–7. The utilization of the services of physicians and hospitals by both public-assistance

Table 9–7
Use of Physicians and Hospitals by Low-Income People, by Health Status and Welfare Eligibility, 1969, Number per Person

	Health Status					
	Public-Assistance Recipients			Other Low-Income People		
Service Used	Good	Average	Poor	Good	Average	Poor
Visits to Physicians	4.09	4.95	7.10	2.69	3.36	5.12
Admissions to hospital	0.14	0.16	0.21	0.09	0.11	0.15
Days in hospital	2.40	2.72	3.47	1.18	1.42	2.04

Source: Adapted from Karen Davis and Roger Reynolds, "The Impact of Medicare and Medicaid on Access to Medical Care," In Richard Rosett (Ed.), *The Role of Health Insurance in the Health Services Sector* (New York: Neale Watson Academic Publications for the National Bureau of Economic Research, 1976), p. 404.

recipients and other low-income people was found to be closely associated with health status (as measured by the number of days of restricted activity and the number of chronic conditions). For every level of health status, public-assistance recipients made greater use of services than others with low incomes. For example, a recipient with average health would visit a physician 50 percent more often and spend nearly twice as many days in the hospital as a nonwelfare recipient with similar health status. By reducing the out-of-pocket cost of care to zero, Medicaid has thus substantially increased utilization among those eligible for Medicaid benefits. In another comparison it was found that public assistance recipients used medical services about as often, on average, as middle-income people with similar health status; but the poor who were not on welfare made use of services to a considerably smaller degree.

Rabin and Albert found that in the Baltimore standard metropolitan statistical area, from June 1968 to May 1969, Medicaid recipients were more likely to visit physicians than other residents of the area.[36] The health problems of Medicaid recipients were also more serious—for example, 37 percent were chronically ill as against 22 percent of the middle- and upper-income people included in the study. Low-income people not covered by Medicaid visited physicians about as frequently as middle- and upper-income people, even though low-income people had more health problems. The study concluded that Medicaid appeared to be successful in attaining its objective of making physician utilization by the indigent more consistent with health needs. Rabin and Albert also found some indication of increased use of preventive services by Medicaid recipients.

A study of low-income persons in New York City indicated that Medicaid did result in some shift in the location or type of care received. By 1970 nearly twelve times as many individuals were receiving their primary care from a private doctor, and nearly 25 percent fewer had no main place of care. However, the majority of persons did not alter the location of their source of health services. The main reason was that even though financial barriers were removed, many preferred other alternatives to using a private physician. Among those who preferred a private doctor but continued to use a clinic or emergency room, such factors as distance, hours of service, need for specialized facilities, and physicians' refusal to accept Medicaid patients were the most important considerations.[37]

In Boston the Medicaid program had a major impact on utilization of dental services by low-income persons. Within a year after the program went into effect, the percentage of respondents reporting a regular source of dental care rose from 64 percent to 76 percent and the percentage of respondents who went to private practitioners increased from 37 percent to 58 percent. Moreover the proportion of clinic users fell from 27 percent to 19 percent.[38]

The Distribution of Medicaid Benefits

Because Medicaid is a federal-state program that allows state governments considerable latitude in determining eligibility, the range and amount of Medicaid benefits, and reimbursement levels of health-care providers, Medicaid benefits differ greatly from state to state.

Medicaid expenditures are concentrated in a few Northern industrial states. In 1979 New York spent 17.5 percent of all Medicaid funds. California, with the second largest program, spent nearly 13 percent. These two states, together with Michigan, Illinois, and Pennsylvania, account for 45 percent of total Medicaid expenditures.[39]

The state distribution of Medicaid funds does not correspond to the prevalence of poverty or sickness. The South, with 45 percent of the nation's poor, receives 22 percent of all combined federal-state Medicaid funds (and 26 percent of federal Medicaid funds).[40]

Differences between states arise because some states cover a greater fraction of their poor population and because some have more comprehensive benefits for eligible Medicaid recipients. Even for those covered by Medicaid, there are wide differences in benefit levels from state to state. Average payments per Medicaid recipient in fiscal 1979 ranged from $538 in Mississippi to $1,474 in Nevada. The national average figure was $950.[41] The aged in Alabama receive services costing Medicaid an average of $1,156 per person, but in Pennsylvania the cost is $3,129 per person.

Part of this variation occurs because not all states cover the medically needy, whose health expenditures typically are higher. However, even for welfare recipients, Medicaid expenditures still vary widely. Annual Medicaid payments in fiscal 1975 per family eligible for AFDC, for instance, averaged $279 in Wyoming and $1,824 in New York, though the national average was $995.[42]

These differences would be of less importance if they actually reflected differences in medical-care prices or statewide differences in morbidity. However, these are not the reason for the differences—benefit patterns are unrelated to health-care needs or the costs of health and medical care.

For example, the average payment for physicians' services in fiscal 1979 was $173 per recipient in Alaska but only $84 in Pennsylvania. In Oregon 12 percent of the state's Medicaid recipients were hospitalized; in Texas and Tennessee, the figures were 24 and 23 percent, respectively.[43] Iowa, Louisiana, and Maryland place few of their elderly in skilled nursing homes, but over half of the elderly Medicaid patients in Connecticut are in nursing homes. Average payments for nursing-home services are less than $1,000 in Louisiana, New Mexico, and Iowa, but more than $4,000 in the District of Columbia, North Carolina, and Alaska.

Medicaid data show large differences in payments by race. (See table

9–8.) These differences are such that the average payment on behalf of whites is nearly double the average payment for nonwhites (primarily blacks). Particularly discouraging is the fact that racial differences in average payment levels under Medicaid appear to be widening. Differences are most extreme in rural Southern and Western areas, where whites receive more than twice the benefits received by blacks.

A nationwide household survey indicates sizable differences in Medicaid benefits between urban and rural areas. Andersen and others found that average Medicaid expenditures (and other minor sources of free care) were $76 per poor child in central cities and $5 per poor child in rural areas. (See table 9–9.) Urban-rural differences also exist for other age groups; benefits for the elderly poor in central cities are twice as large as for those living in rural areas.

Table 9–8
Average Medicaid Payment, per Recipient, Whites and Nonwhites, 1975–1979

Year	Black ($)	White ($)	Ratio Black/White
1975	429	715	0.60
1976	473	795	0.59
1977	554	962	0.58
1978	639	1,101	0.58
1979	740	1,374	0.54

Source: Calculated from data contained in Donald Muse and Darwin Saywer, *The Medicare and Medicaid Data Book, 1981* (Washington, D.C.: U.S. Department of Health and Human Services, 1982), pp. 19 and 25.

Table 9–9
Expenditures per Low-Income Person for Medicaid and All Other Free Personal Health Services, by Age Group and Area of Residence, 1970 ($)

Age	Central City of Standard Metropolitan Statistical Area	Other Urban	Rural
Under 18	76	58	5
18–64	158	83	52
65 and over	54	38	27
All ages	44	43	13

Source: Ronald Andersen et al., *Expenditures for Personal Health Services: National Trends and Variations, 1953–1970*, DHEW Publication no. (HRA)74-3105 (Washington, D.C.: U.S. Department of Health, Education, and Welfare, Health Resources Administration, 1973), p. 52.

Lower medical benefits for rural families to some degree reflect the urban bias of the program. Many of the rural poor simply cannot qualify for Medicaid because they are not included in the narrow eligibility categories established for welfare. Thus only 40 percent of low-income rural persons are elderly or members of single-parent families. The urban poor may also have greater Medicaid participation rates because they tend to be more informed about eligibility for assistance, and also there are more organized groups working on their behalf in urban areas.

The lower benefit levels of rural residents also reflect the lack of medical resources and the greater distance to health care facilities. In most states Medicaid will not pay for services provided by a nurse practitioner or physician's assistant unless a physician is present when medical services are provided. Health professionals other than physicians have helped to increase the supply of health laborpower in rural areas. However, their effectiveness has been limited by supervision requirements and lack of third-party reimbursement under Medicaid. In 1977 the Social Security Act was amended to provide for Medicare and Medicaid reimbursement of rural health clinics. This should assist in paying the salaries of physician's assistants and nurse practitioners who are employed in the clinics.

Transportation is also a significant barrier to medical care in some rural areas. Without special programs to bring patients to medical services or medical services to patients, many of the rural poor, and particularly the aged, are unable to obtain care even if their payment for care is nominal. This accounts in part for the higher death rates, greater incidence of chronic conditions, and more serious disabling conditions among rural as compared to urban people.[44]

Health Services for American Indians

Since 1955 the Public Health Service has operated a comprehensive health care program for Native Americans living on reservations. With few exceptions, reservation Indians are entitled to free medical care if they are one-quarter or more American Indian blood.

The 550,000 reservation-dwelling American Indians comprise the most poverty-stricken minority group in the United States. Their median income is approximately $6,000 a year, or less than one-third the non-Indian median family income. Unemployment in 1980 was 40 percent of the reservation labor force or more than five times larger than the national average.

A marked reduction in American Indian infant mortality and deaths from infectious diseases has occurred since 1955. (See table 9–10.) These statistics indicate the much greater decline in infant, tuberculosis, and gastroenteritis death rates for Indians as compared with blacks and whites

Table 9–10
Infant, Tuberculosis, and Gastroenteritis Death Rates: Reservation Indians, Whites, and Blacks, 1955–1975

Year	Infant Death Rates per 1,000 Live Births			Tuberculosis per 100,000 Population			Gastroenteristis per 100,000 Population		
	Indian	White	Black	Indian	White	Black	Indian	White	Black
1955	61	26.2	51.4	47	7.6	21.7	41	3.6	10.5
1957	57	25.9	50.9	34	6.7	17.3	35	3.7	10.3
1959	50	24.0	47.4	28	4.8	17.2	30	3.8	9.2
1961	44	22.5	40.8	25	3.8	14.0	28	3.7	8.4
1963	40	22.2	41.3	25	3.4	12.8	22	3.9	7.9
1965	37	20.9	40.2	19	2.8	10.9	20	3.7	6.7
1967	30	19.6	35.4	16	2.2	10.1	16	3.7	4.7
1969	26	18.4	31.6	12	1.6	7.2	15	3.9	4.5
1971	23	16.8	30.2	8.2	1.3	6.6	7	3.8	4.4
1973	19.1	15.8	26.2	7.0	1.1	5.2	5.6	—	—
1975	18.1	14.2	24.2	7.9	0.9	4.0	5.2[a]	—	—
Percentage change 1955–1975	−70.3	−45.8	−52.9	−83.2	−88.2	−81.6	−87.3	+0.8[b]	−58[b]

Source: U.S. Public Health Service, *Indian Health Trends and Services, 1974* (Washington, D.C.: U.S. Government Printing Office, 1974), pp. 22 and 24; U.S. Department of Health, Education, and Welfare, *Health Status of Minorities and Low-Income Groups*, DHEW Publication no. (HRA)79-627 (Washington, D.C.: U.S. Government Printing Office, 1979), pp. 50 and 132–133; American Indian Policy Review Commission, *Report on Indian Health, Task Force Six: Indian Health,* Final Report to the American Indian Policy Review Commission (Washington, D.C.: U.S. Government Printing Office, 1976), p. 59.

a Estimated.

b 1955–1971 only.

since that time. Since 1963 the Indian infant-mortality rate has fallen below that of blacks despite blacks' higher economic status and better housing. Perhaps this is because Indians living on reservations have greater access to health services than blacks. The rapid decline in tuberculosis and gastroenteritis mortality rates reflects major improvement in housing and sanitation on the reservations, as well as higher incomes. However, the Indian death rates for the factors enumerated in table 9–10 are still comparable to death rates for whites 10–20 years previously.

While reductions in mortality rates among American Indians from infectious diseases has been encouraging, the *incidence* of many infectious diseases has not declined notably. Morbidity rates from most infectious diseases is far higher than for the non-Indian population. Thus in 1978 an American Indian living on a reservation was 3 times as likely as a non-Indian to contract syphilis, 5 times as likely to contract tuberculosis, 11 times as likely to have rheumatic fever, 4 times as likely to get whooping cough, and 28 times as likely to contract infectious hepatitis.[45] The high incidence of these diseases reflects the continued low socioeconomic status of Indians, their inadequate housing, and the limited health knowledge of the American Indian people.

Urban Indian Health

The Indian who leaves the reservation and moves to an urban location is usually unable to receive medical care from the Indian Health Service. Yet many urban Indians are poor or medically indigent and do not avail themselves of urban health facilities and programs intended for the general population, like Medicaid. Hence serious health problems have arisen among urban Indians, among whom a significantly lower standard of health prevails than among the non-Indian urban population or even reservation Indians.[46] Many urban Indians receive only limited medical assistance or fail to obtain any health services; others appear at hospitals as emergency cases; and some will make costly and time-consuming trips back to their home reservation or community to utilize the free health services provided by the Indian Health Service.

Generally new arrivals to urban areas from the reservations are unfamiliar with existing health facilities and are uncertain as to whether they are eligible to utilize such health institutions. These persons are often reluctant to go to local hospitals because they lack the funds to pay for care, preferring to wait until they have the money to finance a trip to an Indian health facility. By delaying treatment, they risk more serious illness. In addition, American Indians may be reluctant to use existing facilities in cities because of language problems or ignorance of the services available. Health-care facilities in urban areas, whether city, state, or county, have not worked with federal health agencies to assure cooperation in the provision of services, and particularly in identifying and meeting urban Indians' health needs. Moreover these organizations have not even begun to prepare a comprehensive approach to meeting these problems.

Summary

Several studies have documented the strong inverse relationship between income and mortality. Moreover chronic illness is also negatively related to income level. Luft has shown that poor health resulting in disability greatly reduces earnings, with the greatest relative decline occurring for black males.

From the mid 1960s to the mid 1970s, health services utilization of the poor increased considerably. For example, in 1974, those with incomes under $2,000 saw physicians more frequently than any other income group, perhaps because they may had more health problems. The key question is whether the poor still have more *untreated* health conditions than persons in other income groups.

Medicaid is a combined federal-state program for the poor and medically needy. While studies indicate it has increased utilization of health services for the poor, there are many inequities. The program seems to benefit whites as compared to blacks, persons residing in Northern industrial states as compared to the South, and persons living in metropolitan as opposed to rural areas.

The Public Health Service operates a comprehensive health program for American Indians residing on reservations. While considerable progress has been made in reducing infant mortality and the death rate from a number of infectious diseases, morbidity rates for infectious diseases are far higher than for the non-Indian population. Poor housing, poverty, and lack of health education among reservation Indians may account for differences in morbidity rates. Because urban Indians do not have a comprehensive health-care program available to them in cities, they frequently return to the reservation for medical care.

Notes

1. Michael Bradley, *Microeconomics* (Glenview, Ill.: Scott, Foresman, 1980), p. 371.

2. U.S. Department of Commerce, *Statistical Abstract, 1981* (Washington, D.C.: U.S. Government Printing Office, 1981), p. 45.

3. U.S. Department of Commerce, Bureau of the Census, *Money Income and Poverty Status in 1975 of Families and Persons in the United States*, Current Population Reports, Series P-60, nos. 112 and 113 (Washington, D.C.: U.S. Government Printing Office, 1978), pp. 9–11.

4. For estimates of some of the expected benefits, see U.S. Department of Health, Education, and Welfare, Office of the Assistant Secretary (Planning and Evaluation), *Human Investment Programs: Delivery of Health Services for the Poor* (Washington, D.C.: U.S. Government Printing Office, 1967), p. 36.

5. Arthur Okun, *Equality and Efficiency; The Big Tradeoff* (Washington, D.C.: The Brookings Institution, 1975), p. 17.

6. Karen Davis and Cathy Schoen, *Health and the War on Poverty: A Ten-Year Appraisal* (Washington, D.C.: U.S. Government Printing Office, 1978), p.10.

7. See, for example, Evelyn Kitagawa and Philip Hauser, *Differential Mortality in the United States: A Study in Socio-economic Epidemiology* (Cambridge, Mass: Harvard University Press, 1973), pp. 73–139.

8. National Center for Health Statistics, *Socio-economic Characteristics of Deceased Persons, United States, 1962–1963, Deaths* (Washington, D.C.: U.S. Government Printing Office, 1969), p. 21.

9. Kitagawa and Hauser, *Differential Mortality in the United States,* pp. 8–10 and 18.

10. Ibid., pp. 76–77.

11. U.S. Department of Health, Education, and Welfare, *Health Status of Minorities and Low-Income Groups* DHEW Publication no. (HRA) 79-627 (Washington, D.C.: U.S. Government Printing Office, 1979), p. 30.

12. Ibid., pp. 38–39.

13. Davis and Schoen, *Health and the War on* Poverty, p. 35.

14. U.S. Department of Health, Education, and Welfare, *Health Status of Minorities,* p. 49.

15. U.S. Department of Health and Human Services, *Health: United States, 1980*, DHHS Publication no. (PHS)81-1232 (Washington, D.C.: U.S. Department of Health and Human Services, December 1980), p. 44.

16. National Center for Health Statistics, "Edentulous Persons, United States, 1971" Vital and Health Statistics, Series 10, no. 89, DHEW Publication no. (HRA)74-1516, (Washington, D.C.: U.S. Government Printing Office, 1974), pp. 9 and 11.

17. U.S. Department of Health, Education, and Welfare, Health Resources Administration, "Decayed, Missing, and Filled Teeth among Children, United States" Vital and Health Statistics, Series 11, no. 106, DHEW Publication no. (HRA)74-1003 (Washington, D.C.: U.S. Government Printing Office, 1974), p. 13; National Center for Health Statistics, "Decayed, Missing, and Filled Teeth among Youths 12–17 Years, United

States" Vital and Health Statistics, Series 11, no. 144, DHEW Publication no. (HRA)75-1626 (Washington, D.C.: U.S. Government Printing Office, 1974) p. 19.

18. U.S. Department of Health and Human Services, *Health: United States, 1980*, p. 48.

19. Ibid., p. 47.

20. U.S. Department of Health, Education, and Welfare, *Health: United States 1975* (Washington, D.C.: U.S. Department of Health, Education, and Welfare, 1976), p. 309; and National Center for Health Statistics, "Hospital Discharges and Length of Stay: Short-Stay Hospitals, United States, July 1963–June 1964" Vital and Health Statistics, Series 10, no. 30 (Washington, D.C.: U.S. Government Printing Office, 1966), p. 36.

21. U.S. Department of Health, Education, and Welfare, *Health: United States, 1976–1977* (Washington, D.C.: U.S. Department of Health, Education, and Welfare, 1977), p. 213.

22. Paul Flaim, "Persons Not in the Labor Force," Special Labor Force Report, no. 110, U.S. Department of Labor, Bureau of Labor Statistics, reprint from *Monthly Labor Review* 92 (July 1969):11.

23. Herbert S. Parnes et al., *The Pre-Retirement Years: A Longitudinal Study of the Labor Market Experience of Men*, vol. I (Manpower Research Monograph no. 15 (Washington, D.C.: U.S. Government Printing Office, 1970), p. 99.

24. Harold Luft, "The Impact of Poor Health on Earnings," *Review of Economics and Statistics* 57, no 1 (February 1975): 50.

25. Ibid., pp. 51–52.

26. Saad Nagi and Linda Hadley, "Disability, Behavior: Income Change and Motivation to Work," *Industrial and Labor Relations Review* 25, no. 2 (January 1972): 225.

27. P.S Lawrence, "Chronic Illness and Socio-economic Status" in E. Gartley Jaco (Ed.), *Patients, Physicians, and Illness* (Glencoe, Ill.: Free Press, 1948), pp. 38 and 44.

28. Davis and Schoen, *Health and the War on Poverty*, p. 51.

29. Donald Muse and Darwin Sawyer, *Medicare and Medicaid Data Book, 1981* (Washington, D.C.: U.S. Department of Health and Human Services, 1982), p. 270.

30. Davis and Schoen, *Health and the War on Poverty*, p. 53.

31. Council of Economic Advisors, *Economic Report of the President* (Washington, D.C.: U.S. Government Printing Office, February 1974), table 45, p. 168.

32. John Palmer, "Government Growth in Perspective," *Challenge* 19, no. 2 (May-June 1976): 43.

33. U.S. Department of Health, Education, and Welfare, Office of Research and Statistics, *Medical Care Expenditures, Prices, and Costs:*

Background Book, DHEW Publication no. (SSA)75-11909 (Washington, D.C.: U.S. Government Printing Office, 1976), p. 22.

34. Davis and Schoen, *Health and the War on Poverty*, pp. 52–53.

35. Karen Davis and Roger Reynolds, "The Impact of Medicare and Medicaid on Access to Medical Care," in Richard Rosett (Ed.), *The Role of Health Insurance in the Health Services Sector* (New York: Neal Watson Academic Publications for the National Bureau of Economic Research, 1976), pp. 391–425.

36. David Rabin and Mary Albert, "Use of Physician Services by Medicaid Recipients," in Allen D. Spiegel and Simon Podair (Eds.), *Medicaid: Lessons for National Health Insurance* (Rockville, Md.: Aspen Systems Corporation, 1975), pp. 211–212; see also, Thomas Bice, "Medical Care for the Disadvantaged: Report on a Survey of Use of Medical Services in the Baltimore SMSA, 1968–1969" (Baltimore, Md.: John Hopkins University, 1971), processed.

37. Margaret Olendzki, Richard Grann, and Charles Goodrich, "The Impact of Medicaid on Private Care for the Urban Poor," *Medical Care* 10, no. 3 (May-June 1972):204.

38. Dennis Leverett and Anthony Jong, "Variations in Use of Dental Care Facilities by Low-Income White and Black Urban Populations," *Journal of the American Dental Association* 80, no. 1 (January 1970): 139.

39. Muse and Sawyer, *Medicare and Medicaid Data Book*, p. 107.

40. U.S. Department of Health, Education, and Welfare, Health Care Financing Administration, *Medicaid Management Reports, Annual Report, Fiscal Year 1976* (Washington, D.C.: Health Care Financing Administration, n.d.), table 1.

41. Muse and Sayer, *Medicare and Medicaid Data Book*, p. 107.

42. U.S. Department of Health, Education, and Welfare, Health Care Financing Administration, *Data on the Medicaid Program: Eligibility, Services, Expenditures, Fiscal Years 1966–1977* (Washington, D.C.: Institute for Medicaid Management, 1977), p. 83.

43. Muse and Sawyer, *Medicare and Medicaid Data Book*, p. 98.

44. Davis and Schoen, *Health and the War on Poverty*, pp. 81–82.

45. Indian Health Service, *Illness among Indians and Alaska Natives, 1970–1978*, DHEW Publication no. (HSA)79-12040 (Washington, D.C.: U.S. Public Health Service, 1979), pp. 15, 16, 24, and 34.

46. Alan Sorkin, *The Urban American Indian* (Lexington, Mass: Lexington Books, D.C. Heath, 1978), p. 47.

Index

Abel-Smith, Brian, 2
Abortions, need for, 162
Absenteeism: problem of, 20, 130, 134; reduction in, 137
Academic: medicine, 115; training, 63
Accidents: insurance for, 197; problem of, 112–113, 179, 199–200; traffic, 140
Acton, J., 36, 121
Acute care medical attention, 187
Administrative finances and responsibilities, 167–175, 206–207
Administrators, hospital, 13, 17, 62–63, 169
Admissions: discretionary, 177; hospital, 81–82, 86; patient, 81, 88; selectivity, 84, 95
Advertising in medical profession, 17
Africa, 72, 140, 146, 157; East, 68, 70–71; Middle, 68; South, 137; West, 68
Age: adjustment for, 14; death rate by, 98; distribution of, 17, 50; and the elderly, 15, 158, 175–176, 181, 197, 208, 210; factor of, 16, 32–33, 37, 115, 119–120, 174, 195, 202, 207, 213–214; middle years, 21; of population, 86, 89, and poverty, 84, 208, 210; and prime working years, 121; retirement, 119; sixty-five and over, 4–5, 174, 176
Agencies: governmental, 94; health, 172; planning, 129
Agrarian society, 150, 155
Agriculture, U.S. Department of, 195
Agriculture and agricultural activities, 134, 162; income from, 141; production output, 107, 139, subsistence levels of, 120; workforce in, 36, 154
Aid to Families with Dependent Children (AFDC) program, 207–209
Air pollution, problem of, 19, 30, 140
Alabama, 212
Alaska, 212
Albert, Mary, 211
Alcohol: effects of, 30; treatment programs for, 20
Algeria, 153
Allied Health Manpower, 62–66
Ambulatory care, 5
American Association for Labor Legislation, 179
American Hospital Association (AHA), 86
American Indians. See Indians, American
American Medical Association (AMA), 53, 63, 180
Andersen, Ronald, 178, 213; behavioral model, 32–33

Anemia, health problem of, 137
Anesthesia, factor of, 62
Angola, 153
Ansari, 135
Antipoverty programs, instigation of, 182
Anxiety, forms of, 20
Appendectomy, cases of, 9, 12
Apportionment rates, 92
Argentina, 130, 153
Arizona, 100
Arkansas, 207
Armed Services, factor of, 179
Army Corps of Engineers, 107
Arnett, Ross, III, 4n, 6n
Arrow, Kenneth, 18
Arthritis, 200–201
Asia, 72, 157; East, 68, 145; South and Southeast, 145–146
Assistance: cash recipients of, 207, 210; eligibility for, 214; housing, 195; public, 119, 195, 206, 210
Asthma, attacks of, 201
Attitude(s): changes in, 159; mental, 138–139; modern, 147; positive, 141; value of, 93–94, 29–34
Audits, periodic, 93–94
Australia, 1, 3, 130
Austria, 15
Auxiliaries: health, 9, 66–68; midwives, 67; nurses, 66; training of, 68

Baccalaureate medical programs, 65
Bangladesh, 69
Barbados, 157
Barbosa, F. S., 135–136
Bargaining power, use of, 4–5, 96
Battelle Human Affairs Research Center, 173
Becker, Gary, 151
Bed capacity of hospitals, 31, 40, 101–102
Behavioral patterns and models, 29–33, 101
Belgium, 15
Berelson, Bernard, 157
Bertera, Robert, 124
Bias. See Discrimination
Bilsborrow, Richard, 154
Biologic demand, factor of, 48–49
Birthrate(s): changes in, 145; in developing countries, 163; and economic activity, 158–159; and income distribution, 159–161; prevention programs, 147–148; reduction in, 148–150, 162, trends in, 134, 146–147, 154–156
Black ethnic group: health of, 205, 213; jobs

221

open to, 206; males in, 217; mortality rate of, 15
Blindness and vision impairment, 122, 200–201, 207
Blue Cross plans, 6, 31, 90–92, 102, 171, 191
Bolivia, 153
Bond rates, factor of, 114
Borrowing and borrowers, 92, 108, 170
Boston, Massachusetts, 211
Brazil, 138, 153; Northeast, 135–136; Rico Doce Valley in, 137
Breast cancer, problem of, 12
Breitner, Bina, 65
British National Health Service, 14
Broida, 178
Budgets, 170, 185; Congressional, 85; deficits in, 190; departments of, 94–95; federal, 117, 186–187, 190; hospital, 94–95; national, 73, 185; negotiable, 96; operating, 96–97
Bui Dang Ha Doan, 70
Bunionectomy, problem of, 9
Burundi, 69
Burma, 153

California, 212; relative value scale of, 8–9
Campbell, A. A., 119
Canada, 1–3, 15, 71, 74, 112, 130, 134; government of, 185; physicians in, 41
Cancer, incidence of, 12, 107, 117
Capital: borrowed, 92; costs, 93, 109; equipment, 9, 50, 117; expenditures, 92; formation, 151; goods, 85; human, 20, 37, 51, 121, 129, 145, 148, 151, 197; investments, 20, 51, 101–102, 129, 152, 197; and labor, 138; market imperfections, 114; migration of, 138; and operational planning, 94; physical, 129, 151; social overhead, 152
Capitalism, economy of, 108
Capitation: financing, 185; grants, 59; methodology, 13–14, 176, 191; payment levels, 56, 94–96
Cardiovascular disease, 140, 199
Carroll, Marjorie, 4n, 6n
Case-mix differences, factor of, 93, 97–98
Cash-assistance recipients, 207, 210
Catastrophic: costs, 173, 176, 183, 188; coverage, 171; illnesses, 186, 198; protection, 183
Catholicism, factor of, 84
Census, Bureau of the, 195; labor statistics, 8; survey of income and education, 5
Central America, 72
Cerebrovascular diseases, 199
Certificate of Need programs and regulations, 13, 18, 101–103

Ceylon (Sri Lanka), 138, 153
Chad, 130
Chalazion, 9
Chamberlain, 178
Champus public program, 5
Charity patients, public and private, 84, 171
Checkups. See Examinations
Chenery, Hollis B., 153
Cheng, T. H., 16, 135
Childbirth, childhood and children, 113; dental health, 204; labor wage rates, 159; survival hypothesis, 157–158, 163
Chile, 130, 145, 153, 157–159
China, 67, 70, 130, 135, 145–146, 157
Cholecystectomy, 9, 39
Chronic: disequilibrium, 19–21; illness, 75, 169, 217; unemployment, 120
Cigarettes, harmful effects of, 30
Circulatory system, diseases of, 112–113
Cirrhosis of the liver, 199
Claims, financing insurance, 170
Clark, Colin, 152–153, 163
Clinical: laboratories, 83; teaching processes, 65
Clinics, health and visits to, 9, 16, 33, 66, 211, 214
Coale, A. J., 150–151, 163
Coelen, Craig, 100–101
Coinsurance, policy and levels of, 4, 30, 168–169, 175, 181–186
Coleman, John, 3n
Collective bargaining, results of, 4–5
Colombia, 71, 145, 153, 157
Colorado, 101
Commercial health insurance, 6, 180, 191
Committee on the Costs of Medical Care, 180
Communicable diseases, 19
Community: health and workers, 62, 67; hospital revenues, 92; rating, 173; water supplies, 119
Compensation: unemployment, 197; workers', 5, 179, 195
Competition, industrial market, 17–20, 47, 172–173, 185, 187
Comprehensive Health Insurance Plan (CHIP), 186–190
Comprehensive Health Manpower Training Act of 1971, 56
Comptroller General, Office of, 64
Computer industry, influence of, 85
Conference on Trade and Development, 74
Congenital anomalies, problem of, 113
Congress, 183–184, 191; Budget Office of, 85; health messages to, 180
Conly, Gladys, 136
Connecticut, 100, 212
Constraints on modern life, 147

Construction: industrial, 8; of medical
    facilities, 58, 98; school, 56
Consultants and consulting activities, 93
Consumer: behavior, 29−30, 91; demand
    framework, 31; expenditures, 28;
    ignorance, 17−18, 21; incomes, 25, 28;
    prices, 84−85; tastes and preferences,
    25−26
Consumer Price Index (CPI), 8−9, 12, 54,
    196
Consumption: allowance for, 116−117, 124;
    expenditures, 20−21
Contraceptive information, 147−148, 162
Control: disease, 136−139, 141; flood, 107−
    110, 124; government, 101, 186; groups,
    135, 137; hook-worm, 129; malaria, 137−
    138; pollution, 20; population, 148−153;
    smog, 49
Convalescent institutions, 7
Conventional insurance, 177, 179
Cooper, Barbara, 111−113
Co-payments, factor of, 30
Coronary bypass operations, 88
Cost(s): administrative, 167−168, 170, 173,
    175; capital, 93, 109; catastrophic, 173,
    176, 183, 188; construction, 98;
    containment incentives, 94−95; contracts,
    93; control techniques, 94, 97, 172, 187;
    direct and indirect, 116; economic, 111,
    116; of free care, 92; hospital, 4, 81, 90,
    93−94, 97; of inflation, 5, 13; laboratory,
    179; medicaid, 2, 116, 208−210; medical,
    1, 167, 182; mortality, 112; out-of-pocket,
    168, 177, 198, 211; production, 93;
    psychic, 20, 41; resources and services, 8,
    84; teaching, 90−91; of time, 158; training,
    52, 70; unemployment, 173; X-ray, 92
Cost-benefit analysis, 107−115, 118−121,
    148−150
Cost-effectiveness and function studies, 90,
    92, 122−123
Cost-sharing provisos, 181, 183−184
Costa Rica, 133, 136, 153, 157
Council of Economic Advisors, The, 208
Council on Health Manpower, 63
Coverage, insurance scope of, 31−33, 87−90,
    174−175, 207
Credits, tax, 184
Crime prevention, 18−19
Cromwell, Jerry, 40
Cross-subsidization and cross-section
    analysis, 31, 91
Cuba, 157
Cutright, P., 119

Dales, Sophie, 2
Davis, Karen, 36, 40−41, 210

Days of hospital stay, 16, 31, 53, 81−82,
    89−90, 94
Death rate: age, sex or family income, 15,
    122, 134, 145, 154−156, 163, 198;
    gastroenteritis, 214−216; infant, 21,
    199−200, 214−216; premature, 111
Debts, incurment of, 92
Decisions and decision makers, 107, 110, 123;
    and hospitalization, 169; investment, 152;
    public policy, 108
Deductible initial requirements, 4, 173, 175,
    183
Delivery systems, characteristics of, 33
Delphi Panel, influence of, 54
Demand: biologic, 48−49; for commodities,
    28; concept of, 25; consumer, 31; creativity
    effect, 42; curve, 25−26; for health
    services, 29, 32−34; and supply, 13, 45;
    for workers, 45
Demery, Lionel and David, 154
Demographers, profession of, 129, 145
Demography, 32−33; fabric of society, 108;
    household survey, 159; models of, 150;
    population subgroups, 50; transition
    theory of, 145, 154−157, 163
Denison, Edward, 151
Denmark, 15
Densen, Paul, 178
Density: of health workers, 68−70, rural, 69
Dental: benefits, 5; care, 5, 35, 184−185;
    caries, 119; childhood health, 204;
    expenses, 171; school, 9; services, 195,
    202−204
Dental hygienists and technicians, 50, 70
Dentistry and dentists, 7, 57−58, 67;
    advertising by, 17; income by, 9−10; and
    population ratio, 49; productivity of, 50
Dependency, burden of, 154
Depreciation: capital, 37; economic, 180; of
    plant and equipment, 92
Dermatology, study of, 55
Devastation of war, 161
Developed countries, resources of, 15, 50, 70,
    74−75, 130, 145, 147, 152
Developing countries: birthrate in, 163; cost-
    benefit analysis of, 119−121; medical
    auxiliaries in, 66−68; population of, 146;
    problems in, 1, 14, 45, 50, 66, 68, 108,
    116−117, 134 145, 152, 154, 159; society
    of, 156
Diabetes and diabetes melitus, 199−201
Diagnosis and diagnostic mix categories, 9,
    48, 65, 81, 83, 88, 90, 98, 169
Diets, factor of, 136
Digestive system and diseases of,
    112−113, 122, 200
Dingell Bill, 180

Disability: benefits, 176; impact of, 114, 122, 205–210, 217
Disadvantaged groups, 181, 197
Disasters, natural, 117
Discomfort, causes of, 111, 117
Discount rate, 108–109; size of, 114–115
Discrimination: job, 206; racial, 198; urban, 214
Disease(s), 155; agents causing, 130; Cardiovascular, 140, 199; cerebrovascular, 199; chronic, 75; communicable, 19; control of, 136–139, 141; digestive, 112–113, 122; economic cost of, 120; endemic, 138; infectious, 214–217; multiple, 115–116, 124; nervous system, 111; parasitic, 113, 200; prevalence of, 16; prevention of, 180; respiratory, 200; tropical, 75
Disequilibrium, chronic, 19–21
Distribution: age, 17, 50; of benefits, 109, 117–118; drug, 8; of income, 130, 159–161, 163; Medicaid payments, 212, 214; of physicians, 59–62
District of Columbia, 212
Dividends, payment of, 195
Dollar, worth of, 108
Dominican Republic, 153, 157–158
Dozier, 178
Drugs, 11, 111–112; distribution of, 8; payment for, 5; prescription, 12, 15, 17, 184–185; therapy, 39
Duodenal (nonhospitalized) ulcers, 12
Dupuit, J., 107

Earnings and earning power, 113–114; family, 204; full-time income, 117–118; gross, 116; lost, 117; of physicians, 51
Easterlin, Richard, 153
Economic Security, Committee on, 180
Economic Stabilization Program, 9, 11, 101–102, 209
Economists, 114, 129, 145
Economy and economic activities; birthrate effects on, 158–159; capitalistic, 108; costs, 111, 116, 120; depression results, 180; development of, 130–141, 150–151, 154–155; efficiency in, 21; and health, 17–21, 134–135, 167; incentives for, 185; issues and principles in, 17, 45; Korean, 162; morbidity impact, 114; progressive planning, 138, 147; resources, 31, 163; socialistic, 108; welfare effects on, 162
Ecuador, 153
Education, 32, 34, 49, 92, 129, 150; achievements, 135; backgrounds in, 206; compensatory, 19; expenses, 148; formal, 63; general, 67; in labor force,
163; levels of, 13, 66, 199; medical, 20, 54–55, 67, 75–76, 159; opportunities, 156; of parents, 199; professional, 180; programs and services, 90, 107, 147; surveys of, 5
Efficiency: economic, 21; labor, 129; loss in, 14
Egypt, 130, 135, 149, 153, 157, 159
El Salvador, 153, 157
Elasticity; coefficients of, 27; of demand, 88; income, 28–29; price, 27–29, 35, 88
Elderly health status, 15, 158, 175–176, 181, 197, 208, 210
Electronic fetal monitoring, 88
Eligibility: for assistance, 212, 214; Medicaid, 210; restrictions, 209; for welfare, 207–208
Emergency hospital and medical treatment, 55, 81, 204
Emigration, problem of, 45, 72
Empirical studies, 35–36, 42
Employees, part-time and groups of, 86, 173
Employment: insurance, 172; opportunities, 73, 162; rate of, 118; status, 174–175, 182; value of, 115, 158
Enabling components, factor of, 32–33
Endemic diseases, 138
Endocrine diseases, 113
Engel Curve, importance of, 28–30
English, competency in, 57
Enke, Stephen, 117, 148
Entrepreneurs and entrepreneurship, 117
Environment, factor of, 62, 67
Epidemics, problem of, 117, 155
Equipment: capital, 9, 50, 117, 137; changes in, 101; depreciation of, 92; medical, 12; new, 103; and technology, 13; X-ray, 83
Equity, problems of, 168–169
Ethics, professional, 18
Ethnicity, 32, 34
Ethiopia, 66, 69, 138, 153
Europe, 72, 145, 147–148; Eastern, 130, 154; migrants from, 71; postwar, 71; Western, 16, 130, 134, 148, 156, 163
Examinations: physical, 8, 33, 39, 167, 198; X-ray, 168
Exercise, physical, 140
Expenditures: capital, 92; catastrophic, 176, 183, 188; consumer, 28; consumption, 20–21; health-care, 1–3, 111; hospital, 171; in-patient, 171; per-capita, 1; personal care, 4–5; subsidized, 187; welfare, 1, 150
Expenses: dental, 171; educational, 148; hospital, 5; medical, 171; out-of-pocket, 6, 186; of physicians, 174
Experience rating, factor of, 173

Facilities, duplication of, 85
Falk, Isodore S., 49, 178
Families: composition, 32−33, 159, 195; income, 156, 159, 174, 198, 200, 204, 207; poor, 119, 186−188, 204; single-parent, 214; size of, 32−33; two-parent, 197, 208; working, 189
Family nurse practitioners and physicians, 62, 65
Farm: households, 163; operation of, 158−159
Farooq, M., 135
Fatherhood and fathers; education of, 199; unemployed, 207−208
Federal: budget, 117, 186−187, 190; expenditures, 208; funds, 117, 206; government, 3; health programs, 85, 175, 203, 212, 217; research, 117; responsibility, 206−208
Fee-for-service system, 13−14, 88, 91, 176, 179
Fees: physician, 8−9, 41, 111; splitting, 14; standardization of, 8
Fein, Rashi, 50−51
Feldman, Roger, 40
Feldstein, Paul and M., 36, 52
Females: fertility of, 135; in labor force, 154; literacy rate, 161; mortality of, 15; and pregnancy, 184; white, 199
Fertility: decline in, 146−147, 156, 162; in Korea, 162; increase in, 154−155; and mortality relationship, 158; rate of, 135, 160
Fetal monitoring, practice of, 88
Fiji Islands, 157
Finances and financing activities: capitation, 185; governmental, 1; health care, 56, 175; liabilities involved, 91; retrospective, 186; risks, 172−173; third-party, 89
Finland, 3
Flood control measures and insurance, 107−110, 124
Fluoridation methods, 119
Food, 18, 49, 85, 88, 151; fatty, 140; health, 30; prices, 98; stamps, 195; supply of, 155−156
Ford, Gerald, administration of, 57
Ford Foundation, 111
Foreign medical schools and graduates, 54−55, 57, 70−75
Foster, R., 135
France and Francophone countries, 1, 3, 15, 133, 153
Free loaders and free care, cost of, 18, 92
Frejka, Tomas, 147
Fringe benefits, value of, 4, 172−173, 190
Fuchs, Victor, 40−41

Fuel supplies, need for, 85
Funds and funding: borrowed, 92, 170; federal, 117, 206; levels of, 17; matching, 206; public, 18, 122, 148; welfare, 4

Gallstones, problem of, 39
Gambia, 69
Gastroenteritis, 214−216
General: practitioners, 33, 37, 59−60; psychiatry, 55; surgery, 55, 61−62
Genitourinary system, diseases of, 113
Geography: maldistribution of, 50, 63; variations in, 17, 39, 49, 97−98
Germany: Federal Republic of, 3, 71; West, 1, 15, 133
Ghana, 69, 138, 153
Gibson, Robert, 2
Gini index, value of, 131, 133
Goods: capital, 85; output of, 159−160; prices of, 25; and services, 10−11, 30, 85, 89, 197
Government: agencies, 94; controls, 101, 186; financing, 1; health facilities, 14, 120; local, 83−85; monetary policies, 114; role of, 198; subsidies, 19
Graduate Medical Education National Advisory Committee (GMENAC), 54, 75, 159
Graduates of medical schools, 54−57, 70−75
Grants: capitation, 59; matching, 56
Great Britain, 1, 3, 15, 74, 133, 145, 154, 156; National Health Insurance program in, 49
Greece, 15
Green, Laurence, 124
Gross Domestic Produce (GDP), 72
Gross National Product (GNP), 1, 21, 115, 130, 160; loss in, 136; rise in, 2−3, 151−152
Grossman, Michael, 29, 37
Group: control, 135, 137; medical policies, 95, 170, 174−175; minority, 198, 214
Group health insurance, 3, 170, 173, 182
Group practice: comprehensive, 180; formation of, 9, 14; prepaid, 176−179, 187
Guatemala, 67, 153
Gupta, Kanhaya, 154
Gynecology, 62

Haiti, 74, 153
Hansen, W. Lee, 52n
Harbor Act of 1927, 107
Hastings, New Zealand, 119, 178
Hauser, Philip, 199
Headache, discomfort of, 20
Health: agencies, 172; American Indians, 195; auxiliaries, 9, 66−68; barriers, 167; capital, 29, 37; care, 1−3, 12, 30, 111, 120,

175, 186; centers, 14, 62, 67, 203; community, 62, 67; Congressional messages, 180; cost-benefit analysis, 121; economic effects of, 134–135, 167; education, 20, 67; environmental conditions, 62, 67; expenditures, 1–3, 30, 111; facilities, 14, 120; federal sponsored, 14, 85, 120, 175, 180, 197, 203, 212, 217; foods, 30; home, 175; liabilities, 186; ministries of, 129; monetary values, 123; prevention strategies, 119, 123; primary priorities for, 16, 76; and production qualifications, 136–140; professionals, 45, 55–56; programs, 3, 85, 95, 121, 123, 175, 180, 197, 203, 212, 217; public, 119, 217; rural, 120–121; services, 29, 32–34, 50, 120–121, 217; specialists, 129; status variables, 29, 42, 204; teaching, 180; urban, 216–217; workers, 45, 66–70, 120
Health, Education and Welfare, Department of (DHEW), 63, 65, 185
Health Care Financing Administration, 99, 175
Health and Human Service, Department of (DHHS), 185
Health Interview Survey, results of, 41
Health Maintenance Organizations (HMO), 14, 88, 179, 187, 191; costs of, 177
Health Manpower Legislation, 55–59
Health Professions Assistance Act of 1976, 57–59
Health Professions Education Assistance Act of 1963, 56
Health Security Act, 185, 187–190
Health Service Corps: investigators, 178–179; national, 57, 217
Hearing, impairment of, 200–201
Heart disease, conditions of, 116, 200–201
Held, 40
Hemorrhoidectomy, 9
Hepatitis, 216
Herbs and herbalists, function of, 120
Hernia, repair of, 177
Heston, Jean, 49
Historical patterns, influence of, 1
Holahan, J., 40
Holtmann, A. G., 35–36
Home care, 20, 53, 175
Honduras, 133, 153
Hong Kong, 157
Hookworm: control program, 129; infestation, 137
Hoover, E. M., 150–151, 163
Hospitals, 46, 151, 214; administrators, 13, 17, 62–63, 169; admissions, 81–82, 86; budget, 94–95; bed capacity, 31, 40, 101–102, 172; care, 6, 86, 101, 174–175;

community, 92; construction, 101; cost expenditure functions, 4, 81, 90, 93–94, 97, 171; cross-subsidization in, 91; diagnostic services, 81, 204; inflation effect on, 86, 102; in-patient use, 89, 175; length of patient stay, 16, 31, 53, 81–82, 89–90, 94; local and state, 83–85; non-federal, 82–83; non-union, 13; personnel, 13; productivity, 13, 86; proprietary, 83; quality improvements in, 93–94, 171; room rates, 5, 12, 177, 204; services, 20, 176, 210; short stay, 82–83, 204; statistics, 81–83, 102; teaching and nonteaching, 92–93; types of, 83–84; voluntary, 83–85
Households, 19, 147; farm, 163; surveys, 213
Housewives, value of services of, 115, 124
Housing and shelter, 18, 49, 151; assistance, 195; poor, 200, 216
Hsiao, William, 8–9
Human capital: concept of, 20, 37, 51, 121, 129, 145, 148, 151, 197; monetary value, 148; resource development, 124, 161
Humanitarianism, considerations for, 197
Hunter, John, 138
Hydroelectric power plants, 107
Hygienists, medical and dental, 50
Hypertension, problem of, 199–201
Hysterectomy, 39, 177

Iceland, 15
Ignorance, consumer, 17–18, 21
Illegitimacy, stigma of, 119
Illinois, 212
Illness: chronic, 169, 217; incidence of, 167
Immigration, problem of, 57
Immunity, levels of, 130
Income, 31, 66, 124, 195; agricultural, 141, 163; consumer, 25, 28; dental, 9–10; distribution, 130, 145, 159–161, 163; elasticity, 28–29; family, 59, 156, 159, 174, 198, 200, 204, 207; high, 129, 140; inequality, 130; levels, 28, 118, 160; low, 59, 83, 121, 204–206, 211; and mortality rate, 198–202, 217; national, 131; per capita, 21, 40, 87, 130, 141, 148, 151, 154, 156, 160–161, 207; permanent, 36; personal, 89; physicians, 8–9, 37–39, 42; poverty level, 195–196; property, 117; redistribution, 169; real, 87, 152–153; relative, 51; self-employment, 190, 195; survey of, 5; taxes, 170–171, 182, 187; tests, 182
Indemnity, level of, 171–172
Index(es): Gini, 131, 133; health status, 14–17; medical care, 11–12; price, 11, 97

India, 67, 69, 73, 130, 133, 145–147, 150, 153, 157, 159
Indiana, 99–101
Indians, American: health service for, 195, 214–217; infant mortality rate, 214–216; socioeconomic of, 150, 216
Individual practice association, 187
Indonesia, 130, 137, 145, 157
Industrial Revolution, effects of, 156
Industrialized countries, 1, 3, 12, 21, 74, 146, 154–155, 217
Industry and industrialization, aspects of, 8, 140, 156, 162, 172–173, 176–177
Inefficiency, problem of, 88, 93
Infant mortality: American Indians, 214–216; black ethnic group, 15; nonwhite, 199; rate of, 16, 21, 67, 154, 163, 217
Infectious diseases, 108, 214, 216–217
Inflation: cost-push, 5, 13; demand-pull, 13; effect of, 93–94, 109, 196, 208–209; hospital, 86, 102; medical field, 12; pressures of, 10; price, 12, 21
Influenza, 199–200
In-hospital physicians and services, 171, 184
Inland waterways, 107
Innovations and incentives, economic and technical, 138–139, 185
In-patient: admissions, 81; care, 90, 111; expenditures, 171; hospital use, 89, 97, 175; service, 102; treatment, 92
Institutionalization, cost of, 210
Insurance: accident, 197; benefits, 40; claims, 170; commercial, 6, 180, 191; compulsory, 19; conventional, 177, 179; coverage, 31–33, 87–90, 171, 174–175, 207; employment, 172; group, 3, 170, 173, 182; health, 4–7, 12, 21, 30–33, 85, 88, 167–172; hospitalization, 21, 168–169, 175; industry, 6–7; medical, 168, 175; national, 169, 171–172, 181, 184–190; nonprofit, 180; payments, 30; premiums, 6, 170–171; private, 3, 87, 172–175, 182–183; public plans, 175–176; reimbursement, 171–172; risks, 168–169, 181–183; supplementary, 183; third-party, 186–187; voluntary, 4, 18
Intensity, service, 86–89
Interest payments, 92, 108; rates of, 170, 195
Intermediate care facilities, 208
Internal medicine, practice of, 62
International trends in health care, 2–3
Internists, 49, 61; visits by, 37
Investigators, health service, 178–179
Investment: capital, 20, 51, 101–102, 129, 152, 197; decisions, 152; private, 114; medical care, 20–21, 108; physical, 151
Iowa, 212

Iran, 67, 74
Iraq, 69
Ireland, 15
Iron deficiency, problem of, 137
Irrigation, benefits of, 107, 124, 141
Italy, 15
Ivory Coast, 153

Jaffe, F. S., 119
Jamaica, 153, 157
Japan, 16, 134, 156
Job(s): discrimination, 206; open to black ethnic group, 206; opportunities, 159; training, 115, 129
Jones, Lewis, 48–49

Kasarda, 159
Kelly, Narindar, 158
Kennedy, Edward, 185–187, 189–190
Kentucky, 100–101
Kenya, 69, 153
Kerr-Mills Act, 189–190, 206
Khalil, 135
Kitagawa, Evelyn, 199
Klarman, Herbert, 116
Korea, 157, 161–163; fertility decline, 162; economic growth in, 162; South, 74, 130, 145, 153, 163
Kramer, 40
Kuznets, Simon, 153

Labor: child, 159; efficiency, 129; leaders, 6; legislation, 179; market, 46–47, 85, 130; migration, 138; organized, 185; productivity, 135–137; quality of, 150; service, 45; shortage, 49; statistics, 8; supply, 134–135; surplus, 134
Labor force: agricultural, 154; education of, 163; factor of, 20, 134, 137, 140, 173, 205; female, 154; nonfarm, 152; participation rate, 118–120; size of, 151–152, 214
Laboratories, 7, 90, 97; clinical, 83; costs, 179; technicians, 70; tests and testing in, 86, 95, 168–169
Land: reclamation projects, 140; reform programs, 161; usage activities, 107, 117
Language problems, 216
Laos, 69
Latin America, 72, 145, 157; auxiliary nurses in, 66
Lave, Lester, 97
Laws and legislative activities, 180–182; labor, 179; tax, 88, 187
Leadership and leaders, 6
Lee, Roger, 48–49
Leff, Nathanial H., 154
Leisure time. *See* Recreation

Less Developed Countries (LDC), 147, 153, 160, 162
Liability: financial, 91; health, 186; of patients, 183
Licensure, compulsory of physicians, 18
Life: earnings, 118; expectancy, 16, 113, 116, 139; modern, 147; styles, 89, 147
Literacy and literature, 31, 154, 161
Living standards, factor of, 131, 155–156, 162
Loan(s): direct, 57; guarantees, 56; student programs, 56–58
Local government and affairs, 3, 83–85
Location of physicians geographically, 39–40
Long, Russell, 187–190
Lorenz curve, 131
Louisiana, 212
Luft, Harold, 205, 217
Lumbar laminectomy, 9
Luxembourg, 15
Luxury goods, factor of, 28

Macroeconomic: impact of, 108, 145; and population control, 150–153
Major medical benefits, 171–174
Malaria, 108; control programs, 136–138
Malasia, 66, 69, 133, 136, 153, 157
Malawi, 69, 153
Malenbaum, Wilfred, 138–139
Malnutrition, problem of, 120
Management, 85; union, 4
Mandatory health programs, 101
Manheim, 40
Manpower: health, 7–8, 15, 50, 53, 56, 68–70, 75; population ratio, 49–50; problems, 134; projections, 46, 73; requirements, 137
Manufacturing industries, 162
Marine Hospital Service Act of 1798, 179
Marital status and delayed marriages, 32, 34, 162
Market(s): capital, 114; competitive, 17, 47; forces, 21; imperfect, 47, 114; labor, 46–47, 130; prices, 107; return on, 114; wages, 115
Marshall, Alfred, 27
Maryland, 100, 206, 212
Massachusetts, 100
Matching grants, 56
Maternity care, 12
Mauldin, Parker, 157
Mauritius, 157
Maurizi, Alex, 52n
May, 40
McCall, Nelda, 11–12
Measles, 120
Medex program, 64
Medicaid program: benefits, 212–214; in Boston, 211; cost of, 2, 116, 208–210;

eligibility, 210; impact of, 3, 5, 11, 31, 51, 65, 84–87, 121, 172, 175–176, 186–187, 190, 196–197, 203, 206–207, 217; in New York City, 211; payments by race, 212; utilization of, 11, 13, 210
Medical: auxiliaries, 66–68; benefits, 171–174, 214; education, 20, 54–55, 67, 75–76, 159; equipment, 12; expenses, 171; facilities, 58, 98; groups, 95, 170, 174–175; insurance, 168, 175; knowledge, 9; "major" plans, 4, 171, 173–174; profession, 17; resources, 214; risks, 186; schools, 57, 74–75; staff, 84
Medical care: expenditures, 1, 3, 111, 167, 182; investments, 108; price index, 11–12; services, 167; utilization, 202–205, 210
Medicare program, impact of, 3, 5–8, 11, 13, 31, 51, 65, 84–87, 91–93, 102, 121, 172, 175–176, 185–187, 190, 196
Medicine: academic, 115; emergency, 55; organized, 180; scientific, 18
Mejia, Alfonso, 71–72
Melanesia, 68
Menisectomy, 9
Menstrual irregularities, problem of, 39
Mental: ability, 134; attitudes, 138–139; disorders, 107, 113
Metabolic diseases, 113
Metropolitan areas, factor of, 61, 211
Mexico, 133, 138, 147, 153, 157
Michigan, 212
Microeconomic analyses, 108, 145; and population control, 148–150, 153
Middle aged men and women, 21
Middle East geographical area, 134
Midwife Home Visiting Program, 123–124
Midwives, 71; auxiliary, 67
Migration and migrants, 129, 138; from Europe, 71
Mills, Congressman, 185–190, 206
Ministries of Health, responsibilities of, 129, 141
Minnesota, 100
Minority groups, 198, 214. See also specific minority group by name
Mishan, E. J., 121
Mississippi, 212
Mitchell, Janet, 40
Monetary policies, 35, 114, 123, 148
Monopsony, 46–47
Morale and moral issues, 14, 119; hazard references to, 167–168
Morbidity: cost of, 112; economic impact of, 114; factor of, 120, 141, 195; premature, 124; rate of, 16–17, 49, 212, 217
Morocco, 69, 153
Mortality: American Indians, 214–216; of

blacks, 15; costs, 112; decline in, 156; of females, 15; fertility relationships, 158; income effect on, 198–202, 217; of infants, 16, 21, 67, 154, 163, 217; of males, 15; premature, 113, 120, 124, 141; rate of, 14, 147, 161, 195
Mozambique, 153
Murray, Congressman, 180
Musculoskeletal system, 113
Muse, Donald, 213
Mushkin, Selma, 118, 136
Myocardial infarction, 12

National: budgets, 73, 185; income, 131
National Advisory Committee, 54, 75, 159, 178
National Demographic Household Survey, 159
National Health Insurance (NHI), 169, 171–172, 181, 184–190
National Health Service Corps, 49, 57, 217
National Opinion Research Survey of 1970, 36
Native-born and foreign-born health professionals, 15
Natural: disasters, 117; resources, 138
Nebraska, 101
Neoclassical hypotheses, effects of, 37–39
Neoplasms, factor of, 112–113, 199
Nepal, 69, 138
Nervous system, diseases of, 113
Netherlands, The, 3, 15, 133, 145
Netherlands, Antilles, 153
Neurology and neurosurgery, 55, 62
Nevada, 212
New Jersey, 99–101
New Mexico, 212
New York City and State, 60, 99–101, 211–212
Newhouse, Joseph, 35–36, 40, 184
Newman, Jeanne, 158
Nicaragua, 69, 153
Niger, 69
Nigeria, 67, 69, 146–147
Nixon, Richard M., administration of, 186, 190
Nonfarm labor force, 152
Nonfederal hospitals, 82–83
Nonprofit health insurance industry, 4, 84, 180
Nonteaching hospitals, 92–93
Nonunion hospitals, 13
North America, 72
North Carolina, 212
Norway, 15
Nurse(s), 7, 88; aide, 67; auxiliary, 66; baccalaureate programs, 65; care, 95; family, 65; Latin American, 66; manhours, 86, 92; pediatric, 9, 65;

practitioners, 9, 63–65, 75; resource misallocation, 47; scholarships, 59; schools for, 56; wages of, 53
Nursing home facilities, skilled, 20, 175, 184, 198, 208–212
Nutrition programs, effects of, 113, 134, 136–137, 197

Obesity, problem of, 140
Obstetrical cases, 55, 62, 88
Occupation(s): groups, 186; hazards in, 140; sedentary, 140; skilled and unskilled, 32, 34, 51, 162
O'Donoghue, P., 99
Office visits, 39, 53; cost of, 8
Ohio, 206
Oligopsony, 46–47
Olsen, E. D., Jr., 35–36
Omnibus Budget Reconciliation Act of 1981, 59–60
Onchocerciasis in Ghana, 138
On-the-job training, 115, 129
Operations and operating room, surgical, 40–41, 86
Opportunities, 161; cost of, 114–115; educational, 156; employment, 73, 159, 162
Opthalmology, 55
Optometry and optometrists, 7, 58, 60; advertising by, 17
Oregon, 212
Organization of Economic Cooperation and Development (OECD), 15–16
Organized: labor, 185; medicine, 180
Osteopathy, 57–59
Otitis media in children, 12
Out-patients: service care, 90, 184; treatment visits, 53, 81–82, 86, 92, 169, 175, 190
Out-of-pocket costs and payments, 6, 30, 168, 173, 177, 198, 211
Output-per worker, measurement of, 117
Overhead capital, 152

Pacific geographical area, 157
Pain and suffering, 20, 111, 117–118, 124
Pakistan, 71
Pan-American Highway, 136
Panama, 153, 157
Paramedical health workers, 45, 66–70, 120; wages of, 53–54
Paraguay, 153; Eastern, 136, 138
Paraprofessionals, use of, 67
Parasitic diseases, problem of, 108, 113, 130, 200
Parnes, Herbert S., 205
Participation rates of labor force, 118–120
Patient(s): admissions, 88; amenities, 88;

care output for, 93; charity, 84; full-pay, 84; hospital length of stay, 16, 31, 53, 81–82, 89–90, 94–95, 99; liabilities, 183; and personnel ratio, 81; self-pay, 90; turnover, 66; visits to, 64
Pay-back criteria, ability to, 18, 109
Payments: drugs, 5; insurance, 30; interest, 92, 108; levels, 56, 94–96; Medicaid by race, 212; out-of-pocket, 6, 168, 173, 177, 186, 198, 211; patients, 90; physician services, 13–14, 212; public assistance, 195; Social Security, 195; subsidy, 59; third-party, 90, 94; units, 94–96, 102; welfare, 208
Payroll, 81–82; taxes, 185
Pediatrics and pediatricians, 9, 49, 55, 58, 61–63, 65
Pennsylvania, 99–101, 212
Pensions, 195
Per-capita: expenditures, 1; income, 21, 40, 87, 130, 141, 148, 151, 154, 156, 160–161, 207; utilization, 39–41; welfare, 151
Per-diem rates, fixed, 98
Pererra da Costa, D. P., 135–136
Perrott, 178
Perry, Henry, 65
Personal: care expenditures, 4–5; income, 89
Personnel; full-time, 81; health, 45–48, 57, 95; hospital, 13; and patient ratio, 81; primary care, 65; turnover of, 68, 134
Peru, 133, 153
Peurpericum, 113
Pharmacists, 7, 17, 60; registered, 83
Pharmacy, 58; school of, 56
Phelps, Charles, 35–36, 40, 84
Philanthropy, factor of, 84
Philippines, 73–74, 133, 135, 137, 145, 153, 157, 159
Physical: capital, 129, 151; examinations, 8, 33, 39, 167, 198; exercise, 140; investments, 151
Physician(s), 7, 168–169; advertising by, 17; Canadian, 41; distribution of, 59–62; family practice, 62; fees, 8–9, 13–14, 41, 51, 111, 212; hospital, 84; income, 8–9, 37–39, 42, 54; maldistribution of, 39–40, 45; offices, 7, 53; per capita, 31; population ratio, 37–40, 51, 54–55, 60–61, 73; primary care, 49, 59–62; productivity, 9, 75; quality care by, 68; services, 20, 37–39, 171, 176, 184–185, 212; shortage of, 7, 45, 48–50, 55; supply, 9; utilization, 41, 48; visits by, 31, 51, 53, 202, 211
Physicians assistant, 7, 9, 50, 63–65, 75, 214
Pizurki, Helena, 71–72

Plague, The, 155
Planning agencies and services: economic, 129, 138; family, 117, 123, 147, 149, 159–160, 162
Plant facilities, 101; depreciation of, 92; power, 107
Plastic surgery, 55
Pneumonia, 199–200; nonhospitalized, 12
Podiatry and podiatrists, 7, 58, 60
Poison and poisonings, problem of, 113
Policy holders, insurance high-risk, 182, 198
Pollution; air, 19, 30, 140; control, 20
Ponnighaus, J. M., 121
Population: aging of, 86, 89; control, 148–150, 153; dentist ratio, 49; in developing countries, 146; growth, 87, 145, 151–154, 163; health status of, 4, 84, 89; manpower ratio, 49–50; physician ratio, 37–40, 51, 54–55, 60–61, 73; self-sufficient, 172; subgroups socioeconomically, 50; world variables in, 146–147, 150
Positive thinking, medical need for, 141
Post-war Europe, problems of, 71
Poverty: age factor involved, 84, 208, 210; areas of, 15, 198; effects of, 176, 182, 184, 197; housing factor, 200; levels, 195–196, 205, 208; low-income families, 119, 186–188, 201–204; urban, 214
Practitioners: general, 33, 37, 59–60; nurse, 9, 63–65, 75; primary health, 49, 59, 62, 66
Pregnancy, state of, 113, 119, 123, 184, 197 208
Premature: disability, 111; morbidity, 124; mortality, 113, 120, 124, 141
Premiums, insurance levels of, 3, 6, 85, 167, 170–171, 177, 181–182
Prepaid capitation and group practice, 176–179, 181, 187, 191
Prescription drugs, 12, 15, 17, 184–185
Pressures: peer, 14; population, 116–117
Preventive measures and services, 119, 123, 186
Price: consciousness, 28; consumer, 84–85; elasticity, 27, 35, 88; food, 98; indexes, 11–12, 97; inflationary, 12, 21; market, 107; percentage changes in, 27; setters, 30; takers, 30
Primary health care, 16, 49, 59–62, 65–66, 76
Private: charities, 171; diagnostic services, 81, 204; health insurance, 3, 87, 172–175, 182–183; investments, 114; personal care expenditures, 4–5
Production and productivity: agricultural, 107, 139; costs, 93; of dentists, 50; gains

in, 86; health and hospital, 13, 86, 136–
140; labor, 85, 135–137; loss of, 111, 135;
of physicians, 9, 75; wage effect on, 149; of
workers, 20, 136, 141, 150
Professional: education, 180; ethics, 18;
prestige, 39, 84; standards, 49; training,
57, 67
Professionals, medical and health, 17, 45,
55–56, 75, 198, 214
Profit, levels of, 7, 13, 19, 83–84, 175;
maximization, 47
Property, income from, 117
Proprietary hospitals, 83
Prostate problems, 199
Psychiatry, 62; general, 55
Psychic costs, 20, 41
Public: assistance, 119, 195, 206, 210;
charity, 171; funds, 18, 122, 148;
insurance plans, 175–176; policy
decisions, 108; programs, 3, 15, 119, 190,
214, 217; safety, 18; work projects, 107,
110
Public Law, 96–76, 58
Puerto Rico, 157, 159
Purchasing power, variations in, 172–173

Quality: health care, 14, 18, 68, 178–179,
191; hospital improvements, 93–94, 171;
labor products, 31, 150; services, 94–95;
trade-offs, 93
Quantity: demands for, 26–27; maximum,
25–26; of resources, 45, 108; of services,
181

Rabin, David, 211
Race: discrimination by, 198; influence of,
32, 37, 118, 205; Medicaid payments by,
212
Radiology: services, 63, 90, 97; technicians,
70, 84
Rate setting methodology, 94–97, 102;
interest, 170, 195
Reagan, Ronald W., reform policies of, 190
Real income, value of, 87, 152–153
Recessions, effect of, 6, 10, 196
Reclamation projects, land, 140
Recovery hospital rooms, 97
Recreation and leisure time, use of, 28, 107,
158
Redistribution of income, 169
Regression analysis, factor of, 96
Regulations and regulatory commissions, 13,
97
Reidel, 178
Reimbursement: insurance, 171–172;
mechanism, 90–95; third-party, 171–172,
177, 185, 188, 214

Relative income value scale, 8–9, 51
Religion, influence of, 32, 34
Renal disease, problem of, 199
Rent, payment of, 195
Repetto, Robert, 160–161
Research: empirical, 29; federal, 117;
medical, 19; problems of, 30, 93, 115,
119, 129
Researchers, methodology of, 63, 120
Reservation areas for American Indians,
214–216
Resources: allocation of, 17, 21, 117, 208;
economic, 31, 163; human, 124, 161; level
of, 8, 129; medical, 214; nursing, 47;
natural, 138; reallocation of, 85, 138;
scarcity of, 45, 108, 117; use of, 111, 124,
161
Respiratory system, 113, 122, 200
Responsibilities: administrative, 206–208
Retirement and retired persons, 116–117,
119
Revenues, community hospital, 92
Reynolds, Roger, 40, 210
Rheumatic fever, 216
Rhode Island, 207
Rhodesia, 153
Ribicoff, Abraham, 187, 189–190
Rice, Dorothy, 111–113, 115
Rich, William, 160
Risk: financial, 172–173; insurance,
168–169, 181–183; medical, 186;
uncertainty problems of, 109–110
River and Harbor Act, 107
Roback, G. A., 62
Robertson, 178
Roemer, 66
Ronaghy, 67
Room rates in hospitals, 5, 12
Roosevelt, Franklin D., administration of,
180
Rosenzweig, M. R., 159
Rosett, Richard, 210
Royston, Erica, 71–72
Rubella, contagious disease of, 118
Ruderman, Peter, 129
Rural areas, 41, 61, 98, 162–163, 197–198,
217; density of, 69; families in, 214; health
services, 64, 66, 120–121; Medicaid
benefits in, 213
Russell, Louise, 36

Safety precautions, 18
Sanders, B. S., 16
St. Louis, Missouri, 110
St. Lucia, Island of, 135
Salaries, 13–14, 81–82, 181, 195. See also
Wages

Sanitariums, need for, 67
Sanitation: departments, 20; programs, 67, 134, 216
Sardinia, 138
Saywer, Darwin, 213
Schelling, Thomas, 122
Scheffler, R. M., 63
Schistosomiasis, spread of, 130, 135–136, 140–141
Schoenbaum, S. C., 118
Scholarships, 56, 58; nursing, 59
Schonfeld, Hyman, 49
Schools, 151; construction, 56; curriculum in, 56; dental, 9; foreign, 57, 74–75; medical, 55, 73–75; nursing, 56; pharmacy, 56; public, 110; student loan programs, 56–58
Schultz, Theodore, 151
Science and scientists, 18
Scitovsky, Ann, 11–12
Security; economic, 180; social, 150, 176, 180, 206, 214; supplemental income, 207
Sedentary occupations, results of, 140
Self-employment, 5, 8, 173, 181–182, 190–191, 195
Self-sufficiency, state of, 172
Senility, factor of, 198
Senturia, 178
Service(s): changes in, 101; cost of, 10–11, 84; dental, 195, 202–204; educational, 90, 107, 147; and goods, 10–11, 30, 85, 89, 197; health, 29, 32–34, 50–51, 64, 66, 120–121, 167, 217; of housewives, 115, 124; in-hospital physicians, 171, 184; inpatient, 102; intensity, 86, 88–89, 102; nursing home, 20; out-patient, 184; payment for, 13–14, 212; physician, 20, 37–39, 176, 184–185, 210; preventative, 119, 123, 186; quantity of, 181; range of, 83–84, 94–95; rural, 64, 66, 120–121; surgical, 174; treatment facilities, 90; utilization of, 51, 102, 177, 185
Sex; factor of, 16, 32–33, 37, 119, 195; death rate graded by, 198
Shapiro, S., 178
Short-stay hospitals, 82–83, 204
Sick leave, granting of, 169
Sierra Leone, 153
Silverman, L., 97
Simanis, Joseph, 3n
Simon, Julian, 153, 163
Singapore, 157
Singh, S. K., 154
Single-parent families, problem of, 214
Skin diseases, 113
Skolnik, Alfred, 2
Sloan, Frank, 40, 100–101
Smog, control of, 49

Social: groups, 17; measures, 108, 139; overhead capital, 152; progress economically, 147; services, 129, 163; status, 159, 161; structure, 32, 34, 148; welfare, 130–131, 151, 161
Social Security Act, 176, 180, 206, 214; Amendments of 1950 and 1960, 206; payments, 195
Socialism and socialistic countries, 66; economy of, 108
Society: agrarian, 150, 155; benefits to, 18–19; cost to, 2, 116; fabric of, 108, 156; value of, 117, 121, 124
Socioeconomic: disparities, 50, 162; progress, 145–146, 195; status, 206, 216
Sorkin, Alan, 60
South America, 68, 72
South Dakota, 60
South Korea, 74, 130, 145, 153, 163
Soviet Union, 66, 130
Spain, 15
Specialists, health, 33, 84, 129, 168
Sri Lanka, 138, 153, 157
Standard(s): fee, 8; of living, 131, 155–156, 162; professional, 49
Standard Metropolitan Statistical Area (SMSA), 41, 211
Stason, William, 8–9
State programs and responsibilities, 3, 83–85 206–208, 212, 217
Statistics; labor, 8; hospital, 81–83, 102
Steinwald, B., 100–101
Student loan programs, 56–58
Studies and surveys, results of, 5, 35–36, 42, 213
Subsidization and subsidies: health, 187; payments, 59; policy of, 18–19, 56, 182, 198; tax, 171
Subsistence and substitution programs, 28, 120
Suburban geographical areas, 98
Sudan, 69
Suicide, rate of, 199
Sullivan, Daniel, 100–101
Supplemental Security Income (SSI), 207
Supply: and demand conditions, 5, 9, 13, 45–46, 95; of food, 155–156; of labor, 134–135; of services, 102; water, 119, 152
Surgeons, 8, 39, 74–75, 84; general, 61; population ratio, 41
Surgery and surgical procedures, 40–41, 174; general, 5, 55, 95; plastic, 55; rate of, 205; reduction in, 177; Thoracic, 62
Surplus: of labor, 134; of physicians, 9
Survival hypothesis, 157–158, 163
Sweden, 1, 3, 15
Switzerland, 15, 134

Syphilis, problem of, 216
Syria, 153

Taiwan, 153, 157
Tanzania, 135, 153
Tastes and preferences of consumers, 25–26
Taxes: factor of, 181; income, 170–171, 182, 187; laws, 88, 187; payroll, 185; subsidies, 171; treatment, 173
Taylor, Carl, 158
Teaching: clinical, 65; costs, 90–91; health programs, 93, 180; hospitals, 92–93
Technical progress, 67, 132, 138–139
Technicians: dental, 70; laboratory, 70, 84
Technology, 50, 162; developments in, 87–89; expensive, 13; medical, 11, 31; sophisticated, 93
Tennessee, 212
Tests: income, 182; laboratory, 86, 95, 168–169; specialized, 168
Texas, 212
Thailand, 71, 145, 153, 157, 159
Therapeutic procedures and drug therapy, 39, 88
Third-party: insurance, 186–187; financing system, 30, 89; payers, 90, 94; providers, 92
Thirlwall, 152
Thoracic surgery, 62
Time-motion series, value of, 31, 115, 158; waiting, 41
Tobacco, use of, 140
Tobago, 157
Trade-offs, policy of, 93
Traffic accidents, problem of, 140
Training: academic, 63; auxiliary, 68, 70; cost of, 52, 70; health manpower, 39, 56; on-the-job, 115, 129; professional, 57, 67; of skills, 19; technical, 67; time involved, 92
Transition demographic theory, 145, 154–157, 163
Transportation and travel: facilities for, 40–41, 137, 152, 156; factor of, 49, 107, 120, 124, 214
Treatment: alcoholism, 20; in-patient, 92; out-patient, 21, 92, 169, 175, 190; services, 90; and taxation, 173
Trinidad, 157
Tropical diseases, 75
Truman, Harry S., administration of, 4, 180
Tuberculosis, 199, 214–216
Tunis, 153
Tunisia, 157
Turkey, 145, 157; midwives in, 123
Turnover: of patients, 66; of personnel, 68, 134
Two-parent families, 197, 208

Uganda, 153
Underdeveloped countries, 138
Underemployment, problem of, 120
Underwriting losses in insurance, 3
Unemployment and the unemployed: chronic, 120; compensation for, 197, 207–208; factor of, 5–6, 10, 19, 73, 181–182, 191, 195, 214; health costs of, 173; rate of, 113, 118–119, 134, 205
Unions and unionization movement, 4, 13
United Kingdom. See Great Britain
United Nations Conference on Trade and Development, 74
United States, 15, 130
Upper Volta, 130
Urban areas, 41, 61, 75, 98, 120, 162; bias in, 214; health facilities, 216–217; poverty in, 214; renewal efforts, 83, 107, 156;
Urology and Urologists, 55
Uruguay, 153
Utilization: increases in, 102; levels of, 86, 89, 97; medical care, 202–205, 210; per-capita, 39–41; physician, 41, 48; rate of, 30, 111; of services, 51, 102, 177, 185

Vaccination programs, 18–19, 120
Vaginal hysterectomy repair, 9
Venezuela, 69, 157
Veterans' Administration, function of, 5
Veterinarians, 56–60; assistants to, 7
Vietnam, 157; war in, 195
Viruses, problem of, 130
Visitations and visits: clinic, 9, 16; general practitioner, 37; internist, 37; midwife home program, 123–124; office, 8, 39, 53; operating, 86; out-patient, 53, 81–82, 86; patient, 64; physicians, 31, 51, 53, 202, 211; price of, 8
Voluntary: certification, 18; hospitals, 83–85; insurance, 4, 18; programs, 101

Wages: child, 159; levels, 13, 86, 98, 195; nurses, 53; paramedics, 53–54; physicians, 54; productivity effect on, 149; real, 162; of workers, 156
Wagner-Murray-Dingell Bill, 180
Walsh, D. C., 119
Washington, 100–101
Water: development, 49; projects, 107; supply, 119, 152
Weisbrod, Burton A., 116–117, 135
Welfare: economic effects, 162; eligibility for, 207–208; expenditures, 1, 4, 150, 208; food stamps, 195; per-capita, 151; programs, 162, 207, 214; social, 130–131, 151, 161
Wersinger, R. P., 178
West Germany, 1, 15, 133

Western Europe, 16, 130, 134, 156, 163;
 fertility in, 148
Whooping cough, 216
Widows, status of, 208
Williams, 178
Winslow, C. E. A., 136
Wisconsin, 101
Witchdoctors, 120
Wolinsky, Frederic, 178
Women: in labor force, 154; literacy rate of,
 161; middle aged, 21; mortality rate, 15
Workers: auxiliary, 66; compensation, 5,
 156, 179, 195; full-time, 173; health, 45,
 66−70, 120; life-expectancy of, 113, 116;
 part-time, 81; prime age, 121; output
 productivity, 20, 117, 136, 141, 150
Workloads and workforce; agricultural, 36,

154; avoidance of, 118; levels of, 37−40,
 107, 110, 112, 189
World Bank, 160; projections of, 146−148
World Health Organization (WHO), 66, 69
World and international trends: health
 manpower, 68−70; population, 146−147
World War II: ante war years, 70; post war
 years, 3−4, 9, 48, 145, 147, 158
Wright, 135
Wyoming, 212

X-ray diagnostic equipment, 83, 86, 95; costs,
 92; examinations, 168

Zaidan, George, 148−149
Zaire, 153
Zambia, 153; Southern, 120−121

About the Author

Alan L. Sorkin is professor and chairman of the Department of Economics at the University of Maryland, Baltimore County. He also holds appointments in the Department of Epidemiology and Social Medicine of the University of Maryland Medical School and in the Department of International Health of The Johns Hopkins University School of Hygiene and Public Health. He received the Ph.D. in economics from Johns Hopkins in 1966. Dr. Sorkin is the author of *American Indians and Federal Aid* (1971), and of *Education, Unemployment and Economic Growth* (1974), *Health Economics: An Introduction* (1975), *Health Economics in Developing Countries* (1976), *Health Manpower: An Economic Perspective* (1977), *The Urban American Indian* (1978), *The Economics of the Postal System* (1980), and *Economic Aspects of Natural Hazards* (1982), all published by Lexington Books. He has also written a number of articles focusing on the economics of human resources.